Natural Health Care for Your Cat

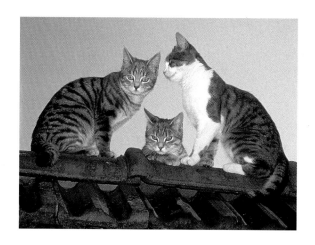

D1551187

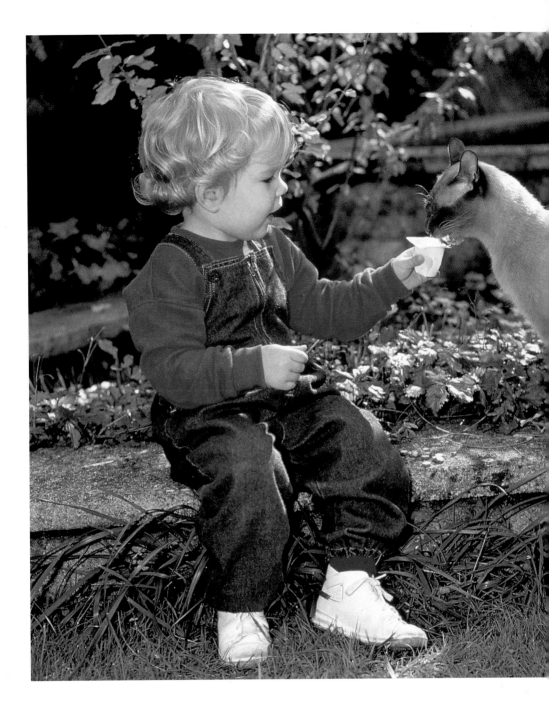

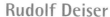

Rudolf Deiser

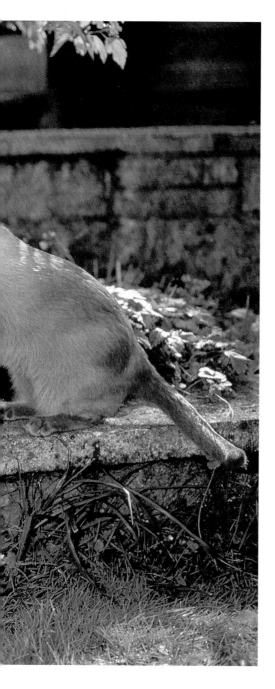

Natural Health Care for Your
Cat

Quick Self-Help Using Homeopathy and Bach Flowers

Color Photography by Monika Wegler

Drawings by György Jankovics

BARRON'S

Contents

What You Should Know About Your Cat

Treating Diseases at Home

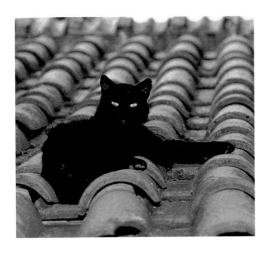

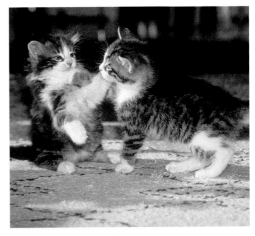

Practical Advice for Cat Owners

Appendix

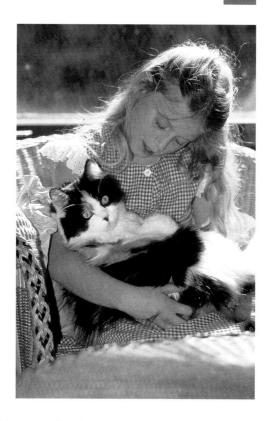

Treating Diseases at Home

What You Should Know About Your Cat

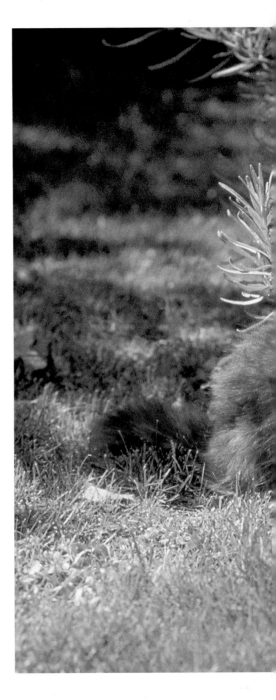

In recent years cats have become ever more popular, and their appeal has now surpassed that of dogs. Feline pets are adored as much at home as abroad.

This does not come as a surprise to cat lovers, who value their cats as much as they appreciate the particular characteristics of this animal. This book will help new cat owners find valuable information on how to properly care for their cat.

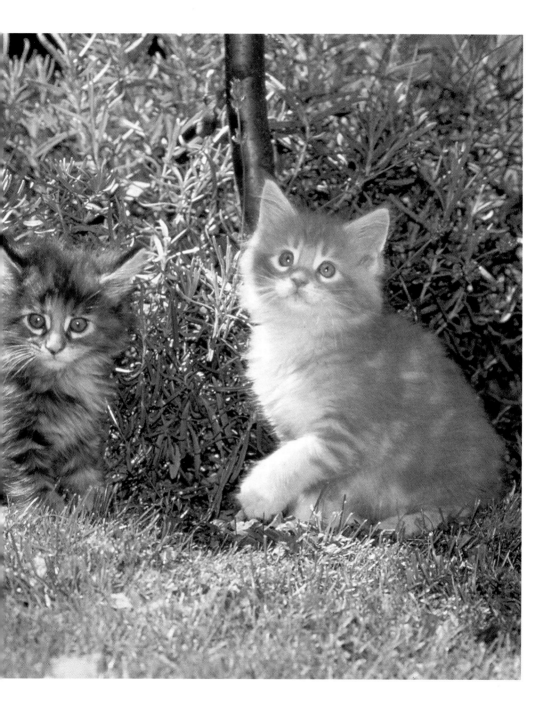

Before You Get a Cat

A cat is a wonderful and entertaining companion, but its ownership goes along with demanding tasks—some of which are not at all pleasant. Before anyone considers owning a cat, they should consider all the consequences in order to avoid later disappointment and anger.

● A cat's average lifespan is 12 to 16 years, but can sometimes be longer. Will you be able to provide consistently for this length of time?

● Cats need attention, regular meals, and extensive care. You will need to make time and effort available whenever it might be needed.

● Cats need space to run and roam—either indoors or outdoors. Indoor cats need a variety of environmental enrichment, such as climbing trees,

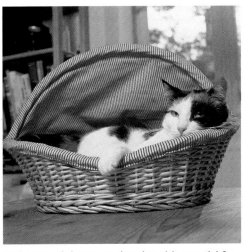

Each cat needs its own resting place. It's essential for quality naps.

Health Check

✓ **Behavior, Fitness**
Lively, alert, curious, playful, affectionate, active, agile

✓ **Physical Condition**
Clean and neat, well-proportioned body structure, muscular, compact, or wiry, slender

✓ **Body Temperature**
38.0°–39. 0°C

✓ **Breathing**
Even, smooth, calm, 20–40 breaths per minute

✓ **Pulse**
Regular, medium strong, well differentiated between pulses, 110–140 per minute

✓ **Weight**
Newborn kittens 80–120 g
Adult females 2.5–4.5 kg
Adult males 3.5–6.5 kg

✓ **Haircoat**
Soft, smooth, shiny, clean

✓ **Skin**
Elastic, dry

✓ **Eyes**
Dry, clear, shiny, (third eyelid not protruding)

✓ **Ears**
Dry, clean, inner surface pale to pale pink

✓ **Nose**
Dry, or moist, velvety smooth, without secretions

✓ **Gums**
Light pink

✓ **Teeth**
White, clean, without deposits

✓ **Anus**
Clean and dry

✓ **Stool**
Dark gray, or brown, formed, but soft

✓ **Urine**
Clear light yellow, without particles or cells

toys, hiding places, and windowsills or viewing spots. Are you ready to recreate your home interior to make a cat feel at home? Is there enough space available?

● Does the rental agreement allow for cats?

● Is anyone in the family allergic to cats?

● Do you know anyone who will care for the cat while you are on vacation or absent? Know this before you get a cat!

There will be costs involved if you decide to own a cat: Spaying or neutering, food, litter and litter boxes, carrying case, vaccinations, and health care expenses. Are you prepared to bear these costs?

Purebred Cat or "Regular" Housecat?

Once you have decided to get a cat, you will have to decide if it is going to be a regular housecat or a purebred cat, such as a Persian, Siamese, Burmese, Abyssinian, or other breed.

Purebreds can cost from $300 up to more than $1000. If a purebread is what you want, you should inquire directly with the breeder association of the particular breed you like. This is the only reliable way to get reputable breeder information. Getting purebred kittens from any other source requires extreme care: You must check the health status thoroughly, and you must insist on detailed information on the pedigree, parents, vaccinations, etc. before you pay for the kitten.

Pointers on Buying a Cat

First, you need to know who the breeder is so that you can find out if the kitten was treated for worms and if it was immunized. Ask whether the animal has been sick, and what type of food it is used to eating. It is important to continue the same food for a while, and slowly change to a

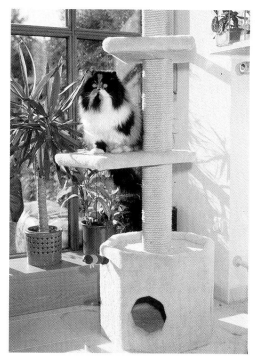

A climbing tree is a welcome entertainment center for indoor cats.

different food. Quick changes in food can cause diarrhea or other problems.

Examine your chosen kitten carefully while it is still with its mother and siblings. All animals should look equally healthy and clean. Follow the health check on page 8. Thereafter you may let your heart make the final decision.

How to Take Care of a Cat

Cats have strongly individualistic characters, and should be treated as such. They will let you know just what they feel like at any one time, be that playing, cuddling, or napping. Trying to force a cat into an unwanted activity will result in aggressive behavior, or in withdrawal. The more you respect the needs of your cat, the more you will be rewarded by affection.

No matter how much you love your cat, remember that you are in charge of creating the appropriate living conditions for it, and this includes its limitations. The most important requirements for a happy cat life are play time, time for cuddles, and a well-balanced, high-quality nutrition (page 12). Equally important are regular health checks (page 16) and adequate preventive care (page 104). It is also important to remove potential sources of danger in order to prevent injury and poisoning (see checklist).

Play

Cats who are kept exclusively indoors require more human interaction and environmental enrichment than outdoor cats. By adding a second cat to a previously single cat household, you can take care of much of the boredom of lonely felines. If you are careful in selecting the companion cat, both cats will be happier and more entertaining.

Kittens learn many of their typical behaviors and maneuvers during youthful play. Later in life

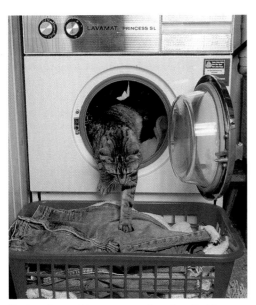

The laundry machine, a cozy resting place that is very dangerous.

The Cat Household

Indoors
✓ Cat basket for napping
✓ Cat carrier, or cage for health care visits
✓ Climbing tree with hiding place and scratch pad
✓ Toys that can't be swallowed
✓ Window seat
✓ Bedding close to a heater (as resting area)
✓ Three food bowls per cat
✓ Litter box and litter
✓ Cat grasses for nibbling

Outdoors
✓ Pet door
✓ Safety screening around balconies
✓ Ladder to and from high balconies

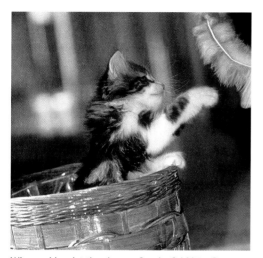

Who could resist the charm of a playful kitten?

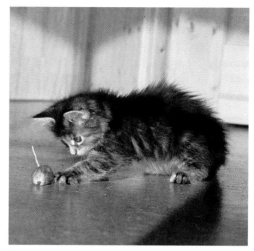

During their play, kittens learn many useful behaviors for their adult lives.

Sources of Danger— Indoors and Outdoors

✓ Hot stove tops, hot pots, open windows

✓ Open laundry machines

✓ Sewing needles

✓ Poisonous and thorny plants

✓ Sliding doors and windows

✓ Plastic bags

✓ Detergents, paints, varnishes, solvents

✓ Kitchen items like blenders, plugged-in iron

✓ Pond, pool, water tanks

✓ Insecticides, pesticides, rodent poisons

✓ Garden tools, open greenhouse, and ladders

✓ Chimneys

this learning is essential for hunting and survival of outdoor living animals. Initially kittens learn from playing with their siblings and mother, but later you need to become the companion for play and learning. You may be as creative as your fantasy allows when it comes to inventing games for you and your cat. A cat's favorite objects include rubber balls, thick knotted string, cardboard rolls from toilet tissue or paper towels, empty cartons, paperbags, and any good hiding place you can create for playing and sleeping. The simplest toys can create great fun.

People who spend time playing with and cuddling their pets tend to live a more stress-free and happy life.

How to Provide the Right Nutrition

For cats, like humans, poor nutrition leads to deficiencies and diseases. There is a wide range of well-balanced cat foods available commercially. This makes good nutrition quite easy. Home-cooked food for your cat must be carefully planned and made with essential ingredients.

Feeding Your Cat the Right Way

Here are some rules regarding the feeding of cats:
● Feed your cat at regular times, even if an occasional hunting expedition yields a mouse as a meal.
● Food should always be fresh, never cold from the refrigerator, old, or stale.
● Cats are carnivores and require food that is high in protein (page 14).

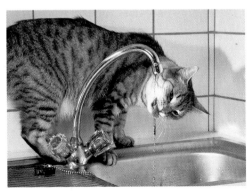

When water is close by, the cat draws near, knowing that it needs this liquid to live.

Important: Dog food does not contain enough protein for cats. As a result, do not feed it to cats because it could lead to deficiency diseases.

● Cats need variety in their meals (page 14). Monotonous diets lead to metabolic disorders.
● Adult cats should receive clean drinking water as their sole fluid consumption.
● Milk contains all the neccessary nutrients for kittens until they are weaned. Subsequently, the digestive system changes in order to adapt to other foods. Milk becomes less easily digestible,

Caloric Intake and Meal Sizes

Age	Number of meals	Amount of canned food (grams per day)	Caloric Requirement (Kcal per kg BW*)
Kittens			
1st week	8–12	(milk)	360
2–3 months	4–5	90	200
4–6 months	3–4	150	150
7–12 months	2	360	120
Older than 1 year	2	400	100
Older than 12 years	3–4	200	80
Castrated males	2	200	80
Pregnant queens	2–3	300–400	100
Nursing queens	3–4	400–600	150
Stud males	2	360	100

*1 Kcal+ 4.184 kilo Joule (kj); kg BW = kilogram body weight.

Milk is appropriate for kittens only until they are weaned.

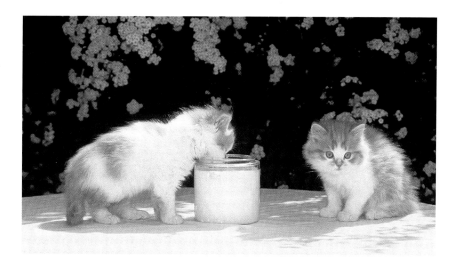

and causes many animals to suffer from diarrhea. Lactose is no longer adequately metabolized.

● Clean the food bowls after each meal with hot water, but *avoid detergents*.

Nutrient Requirements and Meal Sizes

Feline nutrient requirements are determined by several factors: Growth stage, pregnancy, general activity patterns, and sexual cycle or hormonal stages after castration. Nutrition has to fit these parameters (see table). Cats who eat too much and exercise too little become overweight. Neutered/spayed cats and older cats experience this problem more frequently. Try to modify the meals according to the activity stages of your cat. However, be careful, because if you feed too little, the animals turn lean, then skinny, and then, sick from malnutrition.

Young kittens and nursing mothers especially need highly nutritious food. Their nutrient requirements are up to three times as high as at other life stages.

Pregnant cats are fed normal rations during the first weeks of gestation. It is only during the last third of their pregnancy that they require higher nutrient intake.

For how to feed sick cats, see page 106.

Commercial Food or Home-Cooked Meals?

All types of foods have their advantages and disadvantages. Your cat will reward you with good health and affection if you try to find a way to create a varied meal plan incorporating commercial and fresh foods.

Commercial foods are offered in the form of dry kibbles and canned foods. Canned food contains approximately 70 to 80 percent water which just about satisfies the daily fluid intake requirement for a normal cat. However, if the animal mainly eats dry kibbles (10 to 15 percent water content), it is essential that your cat drink sufficient fresh water to maintain the necessary fluids.

Commercial foods have several advantages. They have a long shelf-life, and, as long as they are kept sealed, they do not lose their nutrients. The nutrient compositions are scientifically balanced for your cat's health requirements, and the directions on the label make meal sizes easy to determine. Demands on time and cost are relatively low. Even if you're traveling, it is easy to take along the exact amount of food.

Important: You should not feed dry food exclusively. It is monotonous, and eventually leads to disease. Feed dry food either occasionally, or mixed with canned or fresh meals.

Home-cooked meals also have their advantages and disadvantages. Cats are gourmet eaters who love fresh foods. In addition, many cats have special favorite tastes, which you can accommodate if you prepare the meals at home. Another advantage is that fresh foods are free of chemical preservatives, flavorings, and stabilizers. The latter reduces the number of allergic reactions. Also, you have the option of using parts of your own meals for the cat's menu (e.g., rice, potatoes, vegetables), but you must avoid foods that are spicy, salty, or sweet.

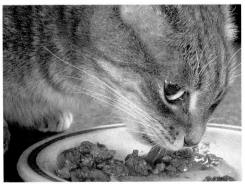

For optimal growth and health cats need a diet rich in meats and high in protein.

Food Composition

If you decide to prepare fresh foods, you need to pay close attention to the balance of protein, carbohydrates, fats, vitamins, minerals, and trace elements. Canned foods are fully balanced foods.

Protein is contained in muscle meats from beef, pork, poultry, and venison, as well as in internal organ meats, fish, milk, and dairy products. Plant proteins are found in soy products and in nuts. Each meal must contain protein to satify the cat's need for amino acids.

Fats are part of the muscle meats, and they may be provided in small quantities in pork lard, or naturally processed oils, like olive oil, thisle oil, or corn oil. Cats can consume an average of 1 oz. (30 g) of fat per day.

Carbohydrates are contained in cereals, rice, potatoes, and pasta. They provide bulk, and quickly accessible energy.

Minerals and trace elements are found in foods such as milk, eggs, and cereals. They are usually fed in adequate amounts.

Vitamins are essential food components which are found in liver, eggs, vegetables, and milk. Vitamin C is produced by the body itself. Too much fish in the diet leads to vitamin E deficiency. Vitamin A must be taken through the diet. In fact,

General Guidelines for Optimal Food Composition

Water	75–80% (yields 20–25% dry substance)
Protein	10–15% (kittens need more)
Fat	9–12%
Carbohydrates	2–4%
Minerals	1%

When a cat licks its paws and washes its face it says in feline language, "I had a satisfying, tasty meal."

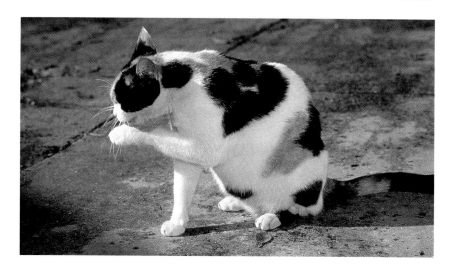

3.5–4 oz. (100–150 g) of liver contain enough vitamin A for one week's requirement. Too much vitamin A leads to bone formation in the vertebral column, causing painful mobility problems.

Important: Minerals, trace elements, and vitamins should be fed as supplements only to nursing queens, and to growing, or sick cats.

Use these guidelines to help plan your cat's daily diet:
● Always cook pork meats to avoid disease transmission (Aujeszky's disease, Toxoplasmosis).
● Uncooked liver works as laxative; cooked liver may constipate.

● Fish must be cooked or fried, and all bones removed carefully.
● Remove all bones from poultry meats, because they can cause severe injuries in the throat and neck. Be careful with frozen poultry, in order to prevent salmonella infection.
● A home-cooked meal should contain approximately 150 grams of meat and/or fish, 1–2 Tbsp. of cooked vegetables, and rice, as well as 1 tsp. of oil, yeast, and/or cottage cheese.

Every cat has particular culinary favorites. As a sign of approval your cat will lick its paws and wash its face after a meal.

Preventive Health Care

Deworming

The main feline worm parasites are tapeworms (page 87), roundworms (page 88), and hookworms. Parasites get into your cat's intestinal tract through contact with feral mice, or through contact with other cats, their fleas, or with their excrement. It is best to have your cat's stool checked for worms regularly.

Indoor cats do not have this problem and they rarely need to be wormed, unless they are fed venison or uncooked pork meats. One annual stool exam is sufficient. Generally, outdoor cats should be wormed twice per year. It is easy to plan it just 1 week before their booster vaccinations. If the stool analysis is positive, a worm treatment will be initiated which must be repeated 2–3 weeks later.

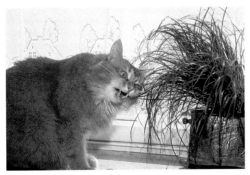

Cats nibble on fresh greens to help regulate their digestion.

Worm Treatment Guide*

Roundworms and Hookworms

	Treatment	Booster Treatment
Kittens	10–14 days	Every 8–10 days until weaned
Adult cats	6 months and older	Every 3–4 months
Nursing cats	10–14 days postpartum	Every 8–10 days at the same time as kittens
Stud males	Breeding season	Every 3–4 months

*Because of the variety of geographical environments it is suggested that you consult your veterinarian at the time of the first vaccination as to the most healthful worm prevention plan.

Tapeworms

In order to fight tapeworm infestation you could either treat your cat monthly with Droncit pills, or you could request a stool analysis every 4 to 8 weeks. Cats sometimes have the segments of this parasite lodged in their fur. There, they present a health hazard for kids or adults who nuzzle the animal affectionately with their faces. Utmost hygiene is imperative to make close human–animal contact safe.

Ectoparasites

Flea and mite infestations (pages 84 and 85) have increased dramatically in recent years. Natural home remedies are available to aid the body's defenses. However, in most cases, you will initially need to rid the animal of the parasite by dipping, spraying, veterinary injections, or medications.

Vaccination Schedule

Combination vaccine, e.g., "Eclipse 4 plus FeLV." This provides protection against: *Feline Leukemia* virus, *Rhinotracheitis* virus, *Calici* virus, *Panleukopenia* virus, and *Chlamydia* Psittaci.

Primary vaccination: 9 weeks of age *or older.*

Second vaccination: 3 to 4 weeks following the primary vaccination.

The first two vaccinations form the primary immunization. Follow with one annual booster vaccination.

For feline infectious peritonitis protection: First FIP vaccination at 16 weeks of age or older, followed by a second vaccination 3 to 4 weeks later.

The same schedule should be followed for older cats with an unknown immunization history.

Rabies vaccination: First vaccination at 3 to 4 months of age. Repeat 1 year later, and then every 3 years or according to local ordinances. For older cats start with two vaccinations 1 year apart, then proceed as above.

Vaccinations

The vaccination plan mentioned above will help prevent infectious diseases, and helps plan health care schedules.

The baseline immunization schedule gives your cat the overall principal protection from the most prevalent infectious diseases. The program consists of a combination of multiple drugs which require multiple boosters in order to achieve full immune protection. The subsequent yearly boosters are, as a rule, combined vaccines in the form of single injections.

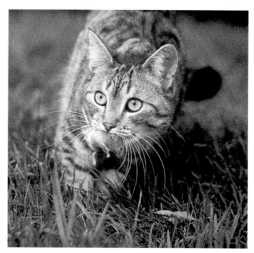

Outdoor cats need to have their stool checked for parasites more frequently because they often come in contact with wild rodents.

What You Should Know About Immunizations

● Despite the generally excellent protection, there are sometimes cases where a vaccination does not work, and the body refuses to produce the intended antibodies.

● After a vaccination the body needs approximately 2 to 4 weeks to build up a full complement of antibodies to fight disease.

● Older cats do not need yearly boosters. Leukemia and FIP, however, are best treated with consistent annual boosters.

● Rabies vaccinations are regulated by local ordinances, depending on the endemic status of the geographical area. While they are recommended for all cats, they are essential for outdoor cats. Foreign travel requires vaccination certification.

● Before your cat can be immunized it should be healthy and free of parasites.

Worrying About Offspring

Cats can get pregnant two to three times each year. Every pregnancy can result in three to seven kittens. The gestation period for cats is 58 to 70 days, and a majority of births occur around the 63rd day.

As a rule, cats deliver their young unassisted, even in their first births. Once labor begins, the first kitten may not be expelled until about 2 to 3 hours later. If the birth of the first kitten is delayed for more than 3 to 4 hours you must get veterinary emergency assistance. The second kitten usually arrives between 15 and 60 minutes later.

The First Weeks of Life

Once the kittens are born, you should prepare

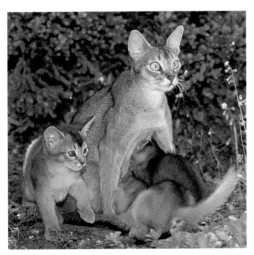

Kittens are nursed by their mother for about 6 weeks.

clean bedding for the mother and her kittens. This will let the mother get a much needed rest. If the environment is cool, you must add a warming pad or a hot water bottle under the kittens' blanket to keep them warm. For the first 8 to 10 days the mother cat will be fully occupied taking care of her blind and deaf kittens. After every feeding, she massages their little bellies with her tongue in order to eliminate stool and urine from their digestive tract. You will need to place the litterbox close by, so that the mother can teach her kittens how to use it properly. The best time to place the kittens in their new home is 12 weeks. Never give a kitten away earlier than 8 weeks. The kittens should be wormed and vaccinated before they change their home.

Raising Orphan Kittens

If the mother cat dies or if there is no milk production to feed the litter, you will need to care for the kittens.

Kittens need to be fed every 3 hours with mother replacement milk, which is available in pet stores. Until you get this product you can use diluted evaporated milk as an emergency substitute. The milk should be kept at 100.5°F (38°C). Although small bottles with nipples are the best choice for feeding milk, droppers, pipettes, or syringes also work well. Follow each feeding session with a light massage of the belly and the anal area, using a moist tissue.

Beginning the fourth week, you can start changing the diet to solid foods. Add small amounts of soft foods at first, decreasing the amount of milk slowly, until the change is complete.

Make sure the kittens are kept warm at all times. During the first 2 weeks, the room temperature should be 80° to 88°F (27° to 30°C). After 3 weeks, 70° to 72°F (20° to 22°C) is sufficient.

Castration (Spaying/Neutering)

As male and female cats near sexual maturity, they develop certain behavioral characteristics that can make them poor human companions. The only solution to this problem is neutering (page 120).

Females are best spayed at about 6 months of age, just before they start their first heat. Males can be castrated as late as 8 to 10 months of age.

Why Should Your Cat Be Spayed/Neutered?

● Neutered cats live a longer and healthier life. They incur less parasitism, have less injuries, and risk less infectious diseases during mating seasons, because they are less likely to have contact with other cats.

● The animal develops a calmer temperament, and it is less likely to stray from home.

● Females will not exhibit their typical seasonal behavior, including urination, nervousness, rolling all over the floor, and nonstop nightly meowing. Such female cats risk a number of uterine health problems if they go through a heat cycle without being mated. The resulting disorders necessitate surgical removal of the entire uterine and ovarian tract.

● Males will not develop spray-marking behavior.

● Cat owners need not worry about the problem of finding homes for their unwanted kittens.

● Intact females tend to stray, especially if they are not used to regular extensive human affection. This results in increased parasitism, weight loss, and high mortality due to infectious diseases.

Prevention and Convalescent Care

Neutering is a surgical procedure performed on a fully anesthetized animal. Most clinics perform the procedure on an ambulatory basis. You can help your cat heal faster, psychologically and

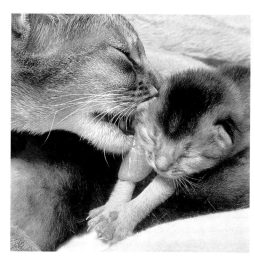

Kittens visibly delight in their mother's affectionate grooming attention.

physically, with the following treatment: 3 days before and 3 days after the surgery administer 1 dose of Arnica 12X twice daily. Then, continue for 7 days, by giving the animal Staphisagria 12X, twice daily.

Hormone Treatment

The heat cycle of a cat can be suppressed by hormone injections. This method should be used only in rare cases, e.g., for the temporary calming of a breeder female. Hormone treatments may lead to pyometra, a suppurative inflammation of the uterus (page 64), which usually results in the removal of the uterus.

Overview of Home Remedies

An increasing number of pet owners are asking for alternative ways to treat their animals effectively and without side effects.

Homeopathy and Bach Flowers are at the top of the list. However, other natural treatment methods are known, and used in animals with equal success. Techniques such as acupuncture and color therapy are finding more and more applications for animals.

Homeopathy: Healing Through Nature

The physician Dr. Samuel Hahnemann (born in 1755 in Meissen, Germany and died in 1843 in Paris) developed the fundamental principle of homeopathic healing 200 years ago: "Like cures like." Hahnemann had performed an experiment on himself in which he ingested China bark, a plant extract which was used then to treat malarial disease. He realized that by ingesting this extract he could induce the same symptoms as would be produced by malaria. The symptoms remained active for hours, and could be reproduced by renewed intake of the substance. He concluded that "a substance that is effective in the treatment of a disease, can cause the characteristic symptoms for that disease in a healthy person." The homeopathic concept of the various symptomatic groups is formed by testing and finding all of the symptoms caused by one homeopathic substance.

In *The Organon,* Hahnemann describes the duties and obligations of a therapeutic practitioner:

Healing is the highest goal of medical treatment; ridding the body quickly, and gently of the disease in its entire spectrum. This process should occur effectively, reliably, and predictably. It should also have an understandable reason for its action by which it can be explained.

Hahnemann emphasized that homeopathy followed the laws of nature, and that its mode of action is as valid for animals as for humans.

Potentizing Homeopathic Remedies

Hahneman formulated the exact methods by which original homeopathic substances are extracted and potentized.

Potentizing substances refers to the method of preparing series of dilutions, by which the preparation is first diluted, then shaken for mixing purposes.

Traditional homeopathy uses *single homeopathic* remedies which contain only one single substance. The original substance must be potentized before it can be administered.

The use of the original denominations of dilutions are generally accepted internationally. "D" (Decima = 10) indicates a dilution of multiples of ten, while "C" (centum = 100) refers to multiples of one hundred. In the United States, however, potencies are increasingly indicated by Roman numerals, e.g., X = 10, C = 100, M = 1000, etc.

Most homeopathic pharmacy services, as well as mail order services, recognize both methods of identification.

For the preparation of a D-series 1 part of the substance is mixed with 9 parts of water (or alcohol, depending on the substance and purpose), it is, then shaken with exactly 10 measured impacts, resulting in a D1 formulation. The next step is prepared as follows: 1 ml of the D1 solution is placed into 9 ml of water (or alcohol), shaken vigorously 10 times, and resulting in a D2 potentized remedy. This series of preparations

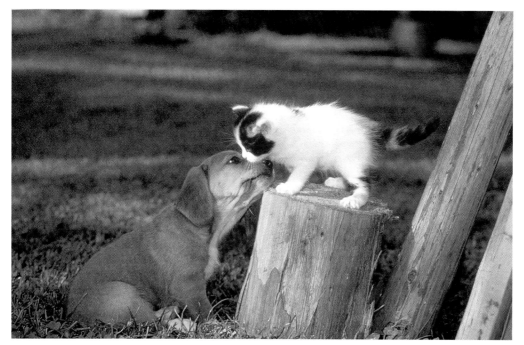

Natural home remedies allow us to positively influence the growth and development of our kittens.

continues to the intended highest dilutions in the D-series.

The C-series involves the identical principle with the exception that the beginning dilution starts with a ratio of 1:99, and it is shaken 100 times at each step.

Homeopathic remedies are divided into groups according to their potency:

● The *lowest concentrations* include potencies up to 12X/12C. These low dilutions are favored for the treatments of animals that were injured in an accident, or that have a purely physical problem.

● 30X/C30 to 200X/200C are the *medium range*. They are the most frequently applied potencies.

● The *highest potencies* start at 1000, which is also coded by "M"(mille = 1000). They extend dilutions up to one million.

● Higher potentized remedies are used to treat chronic disease, and when the animal's psychological balance is involved. This would apply to conditions such as fear of other animals, fear of the dark, or fear of thunder. Behavioral problems would also fall into this group of high potentized remedies.

● 21D (21X) is called the *Avogadro number*. At this dilution it is no longer possible to prove the existence of even an atom of the original substance. The healing effect lies, at this stage, in the form of energy within the liquid that was used to dilute the original substance.

How Do Homeopathic Remedies Work?

Homeopathic remedies stimulate the body's own resources and defense mechanisms to attack and overcome disease. It is the organism itself that initiates and completes the healing process.

Homeopathic remedies do not cause negative side effects, and there is no danger of overdosing. The important factor in the use of homeopathic remedies lies in the regular frequency with which they have to be administered. The concentration is of less importance. For example, 40 globules do not have a stronger effect than 4 globules.

Once the organism is irreparably damaged, homeopathy can only diminish the discomfort, it cannot better the condition.

How to Administer Homeopathic Remedies

As a rule, cats tolerate homeopathic treatments well. There are a variety of forms of administration.
● Place the remedy directly inside the cheek pocket in the mouth. This method is preferred because the substances are absorbed through the mucosal surfaces of the mouth.
● Apply the remedy on the paw of the cat. As the cat licks its paw it will take in the treatment.
● Dissolve the remedy in tea or water.
● Dissolve the remedy in tea or water, and infuse it into the cheek pocket inside the mouth. This widely favored method works especially well on very ill animals. To do this you should dissolve the entire day's dosages of tablets (5), or globules (approx. 20), in 7½ oz. (250 ml) of bottled water or tea. Mix the solution well with a plastic spoon, and infuse the required amount for each administration via a plastic syringe (without needle, of course) inside the cheek pocket (page 104). This method works well even on unconscious cats as well as on cats that are too sick to eat.
● When dealing with a cat that does not want to take the medication, try to use the method that causes the least resistance.

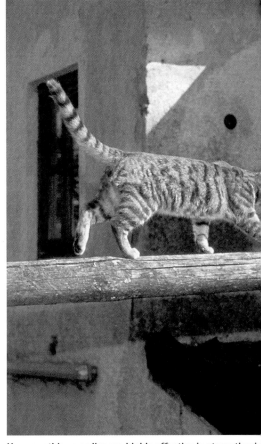

Homeopathic remedies are highly effective in strengthenir

Homeopathic remedies are prepared in a variety of formulations: Tablets, globules, powders, dilutions in alcohol, ampules (for injections and for oral application), suppositories, and ointments.

Tablets and globules are the most useful formulations for treating cats. Alcohol-based formulations should only be used in emergency

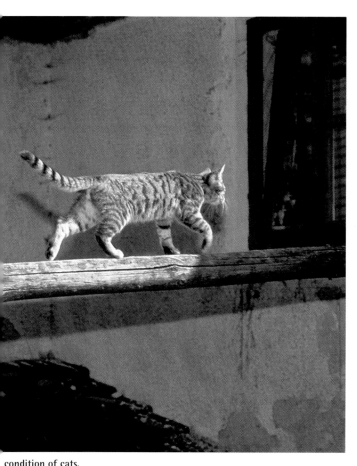
condition of cats.

disease getting worse. This stage is called "primary aggravating stage," and it is considered a positive stage in homeopathic medicine, because it indicates that the chosen substance has stimulated the body to respond. Just as important, however, is the next stage, when a noticeable improvement of the condition has to occur. This improvement must continue smoothly for the treatment to be considered effective. If the latter steps do not occur, the remedy was either wrong or chosen at an incorrect potency. In some cases a remedy will initiate reactions such as a productive cough, a secretion from the nose, or diarrhea. These reactions are not worsening symptoms, but rather signs that the body is trying to purge poisons through these expelled body secretions and is trying to cleanse the affected organs. Another good way to judge the positive process of healing is to watch your cat fall into a calm restful sleep, or to see the animal get up and eat.

There are two ways to select a homeopathic remedy:

● Symptomatic treatment calls for the selection of medications according to specific localized symptoms of disease. This choice will be limited to healing only the specific local symptoms.

● Systemic, or constitutional therapy, considers the entire body, history of illness, behavioral characteristics, etc., before choosing a remedy

situations. These preparations usually cause the cats to salivate excessively, to choke and gag, and to fight the whole treatment vehemently.

How Does the Treatment Work?
During the initial phase right after the first treatment it is not unusual to find the symptoms of

(page 120). This type of treatment will effect an overall change and improvement directed toward full recovery.

Nosodes

Nosodes are homeopathic formulations which are prepared from diseased tissues, metabolic products, or from microorganisms. When these preparations are applied they can be directed at specific causes of disease against which they will initiate the body's own defense reactions. Depending on the type of infection, there are a number of nosodes that are effective in the treatment of cats: Staphylococcinum, Strepto-coccinum, Tuberculinum, Carcinosinum, Psorinum, and Pyrogenium. Nosodes are also a good choice when other homeopathic remedies do not yield the desired effect.

Combination Remedies

Combination remedies have become a major part of the homeopathic treatment pharmacy in veterinary medicine. These formulations combine several remedies, all chosen according to a wider spectrum of similar symptoms that they have in common. The major advantage of these formulations is the ease of selection by lay persons who do not have the extensive and complex education that homeo-pathic practitioners have. Combination remedies can be used by all pet owners with a minimum of basic understanding.

The second advantage of combination remedies is their formulation. They are prepared in the form of *ampules,* containing 2 or 5 ml of liquid. You can either dilute them in drinking water or apply them directly onto the mucosal surface of the mouth inside the cheek using a plastic syringe (without a needle). The contents are usually administered on the first or second day, which prevents any harmful changes of the medication due to long storage or repeated opening.

Bach Flower Therapy

Bach Flower therapy was developed by Dr. Edward Bach, an English physician born in 1886 in the vicinity of Birmingham. Bach studied medicine at the University of Cambridge and then turned to research in bacteriology. He developed the famous seven "Bach Nosodes," which he subsequently used in the treatment of his patients. Soon after, he made the well-known discovery that human patients with similar emotional or psychological disorders respond positively to the same nosodes, regardless of their overall physical conditions. This motivated him to treat increasing numbers of patients by taking their emotional, and psycho-logical patterns into account.

Bach later sold his practice and devoted the rest of his life to finding the most effective natural sources of healing substances. By the time of his death, he had discovered 38 flowers with possible medicinal use. Each of the flowers showed effects on a specific series of psychological conditions which were connected to some physical disorder of the patient.

Rescue Remedy takes a special place in the series of remedies. This is a special mixture of five flower essences: Cherry Plum, Clematis, Impatiens, Rock Rose, and Star of Bethlehem. These drops are administered in circumstances such as shock, injuries, accidents, and similar cases. Rescue creme is also available for the topical treatment of injuries, sprains, contusions, and other acute cases where external remedies can be applied.

Although Edward Bach developed his flower essences originally for human treatments, it was subsequently proved that animals also responded to the active ingredients in the flowers.

How to Use Bach Flowers

You can purchase Bach Flowers in the form of the mother tincture (the original undiluted formu-lation), or you can get a ready-to-use mixture.

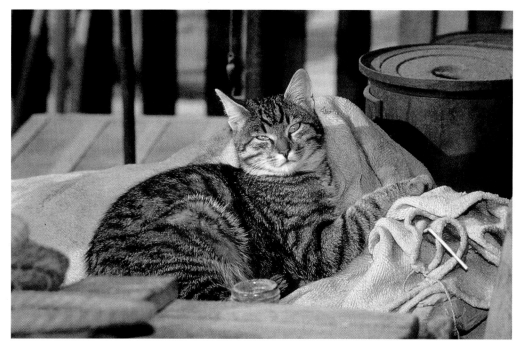

Bach Flower essences are effective for treating psychological problems, like those that occur in the aging cat.

While these products are not yet available in pharmacies in the U.S., there are many specialty health food stores that carry or can order naturopathic remedies. There is also an increasing number of pharmacies that specialize in homeopathic and other holistic remedies. You can also get the remedies through the mail (see appendix for addresses).

As a rule, the Bach Flower essences are prepared in a base of vinegar or alcohol. It is therefore important that, when you order a remedy for your cat, you request that the essence *be formulated in pure water* (bottled spring water is readily available in most supermarkets). Alcohol and vinegar are vehemently resisted by cats.

If you like to prepare your own mixtures, follow these directions: Place two drops from the mother tincture into 1 oz. (30 ml) of water. Always use noncarbonated bottled mineral water. To prepare Rescue drops, you need to take four drops from the mother tincture in 1 oz. (30 ml) of water.

It is customary to mix Bach Flowers as they relate to the symptoms of the disease. Bach stated, however, that mixtures up to five essences can be used effectively.

How to Administer Bach Flower Treatments

Here are some proven methods for administering Bach Flower treatments to cats:

● Use a dropper to place two drops of the remedy directly into the mouth

● Mix five drops into the food or into the drinking water

● Put a few drops on the cat's paws. When the cat grooms itself it will absorb the remedy.

Visiting a Veterinarian Trained in Holistic Techniques

Soon after you acquire a new kitten, you will ask yourself what you are going to do if the animal gets sick. Immunizations are usually the reason for a first encounter with a veterinarian. Older cats will have their regular veterinary visits to receive booster shots, and to check their stool for parasites.

No matter how well you provide for your cat, the animal could get sick one day, and it is a good idea to be prepared for a visit to a health care practitioner's office. We have prepared a checklist as a guide for you.

Important: The more severe the illness appears to you, the sooner you should call for an appointment.

Preparing for the Visit
A visit to a veterinarian is as stressful for the owner as it is for the cat. Here are some tips to help alleviate some of the difficulties:

● Always transport the cat in a carrier or basket that is familiar to the animal. If you plan the visit several days ahead of time, you can place the carrier in the room a few days before the appointment to give the cat time to get used to it.

● Keep the cat safely secured inside the container during the trip to the office as well as in the waiting room. This will prevent unplanned escapes and interactions with other animals. Keep the cat inside the cage when you go into the examination

The veterinarian checks the ears for any changes or abnormalities.

Questions For An Office Visit

✓ How long has the cat been less active or alert?

✓ Have you noticed symptoms such as nasal discharge, watery eyes, bad breath, vomiting, diarrhea, loss of appetite, or lameness?

✓ Are any of the orifices encrusted or caked with moist or dry secretions, or fecal matter?

✓ What is the body temperature?

✓ Do you know the pulse rate?

✓ Did you notice any change in the way the cat is using its litterbox?

room. Remove the cat from the carrier only when it is time for the examination.

● Tell the practitioner what you have observed, and what your concerns are.

● Never yell or scream at a cat, and never use a heavy-handed restraint technique. The animal will only know to react with panic and desperate fight or flight behavior.

● Keep close body contact with the animal throughout the examination; speak in a calming low voice, and stroke the cat lovingly. Only in this way will your cat tolerate treatments, and even injections.

Surgeries

Veterinary visits are sometimes planned for surgical procedures that require anesthesia such as the removal of tooth tartar, teeth extractions, spaying or neutering, etc. The veterinarian will instruct you regarding the pre- and postsurgical care. In addition you should follow these helpful steps:

● To strengthen your cat's overall condition you should treat it 3 days before and 3 days after the surgery as follows: Administer 5 globules of Arnica 12X twice daily. By following this program, your cat will better tolerate the surgery and the anesthetic drugs.

● Take away all foods on the day prior to the surgery. If a cat vomits during surgery it can choke and die.

● Keep the cat indoors at least 1 or 2 days prior to the surgery. Cats have a way of sensing special plans, and they disappear before you know it. Should this happen, call the veterinarian immediately so that you can avoid paying for costly surgical preparations.

● If your cat has a routine surgery, you can usually take it home the same day. Place the animal carefully in its basket, and locate the basket in a warm and quiet room. If the surrounding is

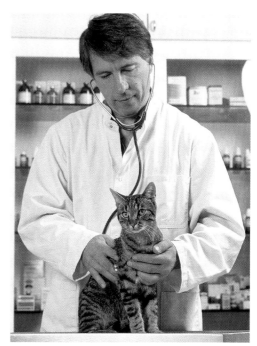

The veterinarian uses a stethoscope to check the chest area for signs of respiratory diseases.

cool, place a hot water bottle under a towel inside the basket. Check the mouth to ensure that there is no vomited material lodged inside and to verify the animal's regular uninhibited breathing. Do not bother the animal while it is waking up. However, cats should always be 95 to 100 percent recovered from anesthesia before taking them home from the veterinary clinic.

● On the day of surgery the cat should get water only. Food may be offered on the second day, but many cats do not want to eat for a few days.

● The stitches are commonly removed 8 to 10 days after the surgery. This is not a painful procedure, and most cats tolerate it without anesthesia.

Treating Diseases at Home

All cat lovers enjoy seeing a healthy, well-adjusted cat that is curious, alert, and affectionate. However, cats do get ill occasionally. When this happens, consult your veterinarian and let him or her help you discern whether an office visit is needed, or whether the cat can be treated at home. The following pages will teach you how to recognize diseases quickly and reliably. This will spare your animal many stressful trips to a veterinarian's office. In addition, cats benefit greatly from the chance of remaining in their familiar environment, and the owner's tender loving care speeds the recovery from an illness.

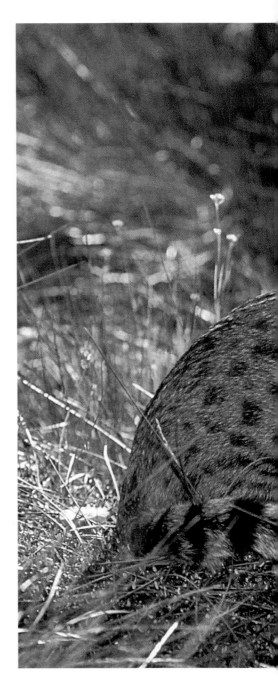

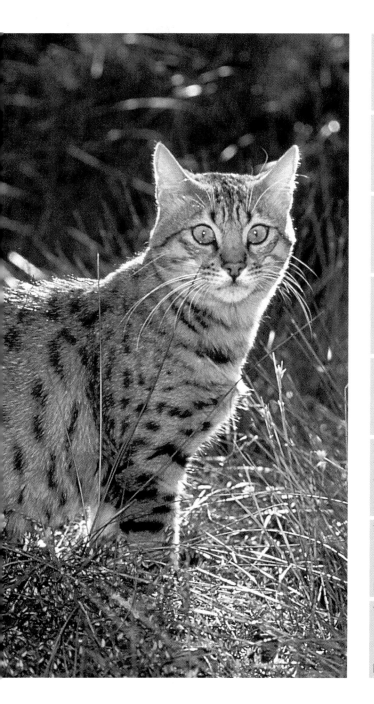

Symptoms	Potential Causes That Can Be Treated at Home	Symptoms That Are Warning Signals
Weight loss	Mating season, increased physical activities	Vomiting, diarrhea, mouth odor, anemia
Loss of appetite	Cat eats at neighbor's house, catches mice, does not like food	Salivation, diarrhea, vomiting, fever
Shortness of breath	Foreign body (food particle or splinter) lodged in the throat	Fever, coughing, sneezing, abdominal labored breathing, choking
Distended abdomen	Too much food, bloating, change of food, obesity, pregnancy	Pain, vomiting, stool retention, intestinal growling noises, shortness of breath, vaginal secretions
Diarrhea	Food changed or spoiled, eats too fast, lactose intolerance	Fever, vomiting, watery-pale, bloody or foaming diarrhea, evidence of worms
Vomiting	Overeating, shedding hair, travel sickness	Diarrhea, vomiting, pale mucosals, tight abdomen, pain
Food refusal	Overfeeding, food too hot or too cold, unfamiliar with food	Salivation, mouth odor, fever, apathy
Overeating	Fasted on prior day, gets too little food, roams at night, food envy	Third eyelid prolapsed, weight loss, drinks too much liquid
Hair loss	Shedding season	Restlessness, itching, worms in stool
Increased urination	Sprays urine, drank too much liquids, nervous prior to giving birth	Weight loss, bloody urine, painful belly, vaginal secretions
Urine retention	Cold season, roams too much	Full belly (hard and painful) apathy, fever

Differential Diagnosis	Description of the Diseases and Treatments
Chronic gastroenteritis	Pages 52–53
Viral infections	Page 92
Endoparasitism	Pages 87–89
Gingivitis	Page 39
Viral or bacterial infections	Pages 90–97
Diseases of the liver, kidney, or pancreas	Pages 57, 59, 76
Internal injuries following an accident—Immediate professional help required!	
Tumors	Page 74
Feline Respiratory Complex (FRC)	Page 90
Laryngitis	Page 45
Pneumonia	Page 47
Intestinal occlusion—Go to a veterinary emergency clinic immediately!	
Constipation, gastritis, and/or enteritis	Pages 51–52, 55
Kidney failure, urine retention	Page 59
Birthing complications—Immediate professional help required!	
FIP	Page 93
(Gastro-)enteritis	Page 53
Pancreatitis	Page 76
Liver disease	Page 57
Intestinal parasitism	Pages 87–89
Viral infections (Panleukopenia, leukemia)	Page 92
Gastroenteritis	Pages 52–53
Foreign body—Immediate professional help required!	
Parasitism	Pages 84–89
Gingivitis	Page 39
Foreign body in the mouth—Immediate professional help required!	
Panleukopenia	Page 92
Disorders of the pancreas, thyroid, and other glands	Pages 75–76
Parasitism	Pages 84–89
Pathological alopecia, fungal infection	Pages 71, 96
Intestinal parasites	Pages 87–89
Poisoning	Page 110
Pancreatitis, diabetes	Page 76
Nephritis, cystitis	Pages 59, 62
Pyometra	Page 64
Kidney failure—Immediate professional help required!	
Bladder stones	Page 63

Symptoms	Potential Causes That Can Be Treated at Home	Symptoms That Are Warning Signals
Skin rashes	Circumscribed local area, cat scratches occasionally, flea bites, too much dry food	Hair loss, itching, reddening, dandruff
Cough	Food particle lodged, gagging, choking, regurgitates grass and hair	Vomiting, labored breathing, eye inflammation, salivation, fever
Itching around ear	Minor reddening of the inner ear, bite wound, tick	Secretion, reddening, swelling
Lameness	Minor–medium severity: sprain, hair clumping between the foot pads	Severe lameness: Abnormal leg positioning, foreign body in the foot, injury
Increased licking of skin, or genitals	Normal fur grooming, ectoparasites, in heat (rolly), impending delivery, insect bite	Hair loss, itching, severe parasitism, emaciation, discharge
Mouth odors	Uniform diet (fish)	Salivation, food refusal, gagging
Sneezing	Dust, pollen, foreign body in the nasal orifice	Nasal cold symptoms, nasal secret, fever, teary eyes, lack of appetite
Salivation	Foreign body, car sickness, teething	Mouth odor, food refusal, cramps, difficulties swallowing
Drinking too much	Warm weather, too much dry food	Large formed stool, frequent urina, overeating, vaginal discharge
Localized enlargement	Blistering, inflammatory swelling due to injury	Warm and painful to touch, hard, increases in size, secretions
Constipation	Too much dry food or bones, seasonal shedding	Tight belly, pain, quickening of heart and pulse rates
Unsuccessful defecation or urination	Caked anal deposits, constipation due to shedding, impending birth	Apathy, restlessness, pain, bloody discharge

Differential Diagnosis	Description of the Diseases and Treatments
Eczema	Page 72
Ectoparasites, skin fungus	Pages 84–86, 96
Liver disease	Page 57
Laryngitis/bronchitis	Pages 45, 46
Feline Respiretory Complex (FRC)	Page 90
Foreign body in larynx—Immediate professional help required!	
Otitis externa, hematoma	Pages 37, 38
Leg sprain	Page 78
Fracture ·	Page 80
Phlegmon, arthritis	Pages 69, 79
Skin rash: eczema, ringworm	Pages 72, 96
Pyometra	Page 64
Dystocia—Immediate professional help required!	
Rotting odor: gingivitis, tartar, bad tooth	Pages 39, 41
Sweet odor: Kidney disease	Page 59
Colds, FRC	Pages 45, 90
Gingivitis	Page 39
Foreign body—Immediate professional help required!	
Rabies—Immediate professional help required!	
Poisoning	Page 110
Pancreatitis, diabetes	Page 76
Nephritis	Page 59
Pyometra	Page 64
Abscess	Page 68
Tumor	Page 74
Hematoma (blood cyst)	Page 38
Intestinal occlusion—Immediate professional help required!	
Intestinal tumor—Immediate professional help required!	
Endoparasites	Pages 87–89
Bladder stones	Page 63
Constipation	Page 55
Dystocia—Immediate professional help required!	
Lameness	Page 81

Diseases of the Head and Neck

Head injuries result in severe limitations of feline behavioral patterns because the eyes, nose, and mouth are essential for hunting prey. Caring for your cat should include thorough scrutiny of this area to find any early signs of inflammation. The head area requires exceptional care in the way it is treated. When serious problems arise you should not hesitate to take your cat to a veterinarian.

The checklist on page 8 will help you recognize healthy eyes and ears.

Conjunctivitis

Conjunctivitis is an inflammation of the mucosal lining of the eye. There are as many incidents of this problem as there are causes.

Symptoms
Tearing eyes are the first sign of conjunctivitis. The reddened swollen mucosal tissue irritates the eye. Itching frequently joins the symptoms, which causes the cat to scratch the affected eye, making the condition worse. Lids may swell with edema (page 120), until the eye is shut. Light sensitivity (squinting) and pain follow as part of the problem.

Persian, and other exotic cats (especially breeds with short flattened faces), suffer frequently from watery eyes.

Causes
If the inflammation is restricted to one eye only, it is most commonly due to an injury from a branch or other foreign object. It could also be caused by irritations from small particles like grains or pollen. Drafts and inflammation of the tear ducts could also be the cause.

If both eyes are affected, the cause is usually a viral infection (page 90). Bacterial infections (e.g., Chlamydia) or allergic reactions may also be possible causes.

Self-Help
For the external treatment of injuries in the area of the eyes you should use Calendula or Traumeel ointment. To cleanse the eye, apply Euphrasia, a calmant solution. Mix the original essence from the mother tincture with boiled water at a ratio of 1:10 (e.g., 10 ml Euphrasia with 100 ml water). Clean the eye by dipping a lint-free tissue in the solution (be sure to warm the solution to body temperature before using it). Both treatments may be repeated several times each day.

Dab the teary streaks along the sides of the nose with a dry soft tissue.

● **Homeopathic Single Remedy**
Euphrasia 12X is indicated for cases of conjunctivitis where heavy secretion, tearing, swollen lids, and nasal congestion are apparent.

Use Pulsatilla 12X if the secretions are discolored, greenish or yellow, and the lids are caked and swollen.

● **Bach Flowers**

Symptoms	Treatment
Psychological trauma	Star of Bethlehem
Over-sensitive, allergic	Beech, Crab Apple, Willow
Runny nose, sneezing	Crab Apple, Hornbeam
Lethargic, apathetic	Wild Rose

● Combination Remedies

For the treatment of inflammation of the eyes use Oculoheel tablets; if there is pus in the secretion, use Mercurius Heel tablets. If the lesion is due to an injury, give the cat Traumeel tablets. The latter may be combined with the other medications.

For dosages of all remedies see inside front cover.

When to Seek Professional Help

Seek professional help in the following cases: (1) severe eye inflammation, (2) when your home treatments are not effective, and (3) if the animal shows general symptoms suggestive of pneumonitis.

What Are the Treatment Options?

The veterinarian is going to place a few drops of local anesthetic into the eyes, which allows examination and removal of any foreign objects. If a viral infection is suspected the cat will receive a general treatment; if a bacterial infection seems to be the cause, an antibiotic susceptibility test will be performed (page 120).

Prevention and Convalescent Care

Cats that are immunized against viral respiratory diseases [such as feline respiratory complex (FRC)] are much more resistant against eye infections. If your cat tends to have watery eyes it is a good idea to treat the animal prophylactically with Euphrasia drops. This is especially true for outdoor cats during the winter and fall.

Breed Dispositions

Persian breeds are more inclined to eye problems because of the abnormal structure of their heads.

Corneal Injuries

The transparent front part of the eye is called the cornea. Keratitis is an inflammation of the cornea. Injuries and irritations of the cornea are very disturbing to cats because their vision is severely limited. The condition is painful, especially if allowed to progress to corneal ulceration.

Symptoms

The cat is very sensitive to light (squinting), squeezes its eyes shut, and seeks dark hiding places. The normally clear cornea appear opaque and irregular. If the condition advances ulceration may occur.

Causes

The most common causes are fights between territorial cats, especially during the mating season. There are also irritations by small foreign objects such as grains, pollen, or twigs. Once the cornea is scratched, an infection by Chlamydia or by other bacteria is quick to follow, unless the condition is treated immediately.

If the animal suffers from cat flu (FRC), it is not infrequent that a conjunctivitis will develop into a keratitis.

Self-Help

External treatment is the same as for conjunctivitis (previous page).

● Homeopathic Single Remedy

As in the case of all injuries, treat the cat first with Arnica 12X. If the condition is highly acute repeat the application every 15 minutes.

Hepar sulfuris 12X is indicated if you notice that the cat reacts in pain to your touch, or if there is pus in the eye secretion. Continue the treatment until the pain has subsided. Sometimes the condition turns into a chronic stage with a greenish discolored discharge. Treat this stage with Mercuris 12X.

● **Bach Flowers**
Rescue Remedy is indicated if your cat experiences shock from the injury. Treat the light sensitivity with Mimulus.

● **Combination Remedies**
Indicated are Oculoheel, or Mercurius-Heel, combined with Traumeel (page 35).

When to Get Professional Help
Corneal injury as well as corneal ulcerations need to be treated by a veterinarian.

What Are the Treatment Options?
In cases of severe corneal ulceration a veterinarian needs to anesthetize the cat, and sew the eyelids shut in order to permit unhindered healing. This is called a "conjunctival apron." After 10 to 14 days the stitches are removed to evaluate the healing progress.

Prevention and Convalescent Care
Injuries are part of a roaming cat's life. If you have a tom cat who frequently comes home with wounds, you should have the animal castrated (page 19). Keep the vaccinations up to date because they can prevent the majority of viral infections (page 17). For the postsurgical support of an eye operation the veterinarian will advise you.

Eversion of the Third Eyelid

The third eyelid (nictitating membrane) is not apparent in a healthy cat. It is located in the corner close to the nose, and is covered by the upper and lower eyelids.

Symptoms
The white membrane swells, until it protrudes over part or over all of the eye's surface, giving it the appearance of a white fur cover. This can occur in one or both eyes.

Causes
Injuries most commonly cause a unilateral eversion of the nictitating membrane. A punch or hit can damage the nerves in this area, causing the prolapse.

When both eyes are affected the cause is usually a general disease caused either by severe worm infestation, gastroenteritis, or a viral infection such as cat flu.

Psychological stress, like a change in the familiar environment, can also cause a partial eversion of the third eyelid.

Self-Help
When you treat an injury, follow the directions on page 34 for the administration of Euphrasia.

Important: If you know that a foreign object is the cause of the injury, do not treat the cat with a topical medication. Otherwise, you will aggravate the condition.

● **Homeopathic Single Remedy**
Administer Arnica 12X, until the eye looks better. If you notice much edematous swelling, use Apis 12X for a few days instead of the Arnica.

● **Bach Flowers**

Symptoms	Treatment
The condition follows a change in the environment	Walnut
It appears following an injury and edema	Star of Bethlehem
The cat has worms	Crab Apple

| It is associated with a flu, or allergies | Crab Apple, Hornbeam |
| The cat is hypersensitive | Crab Apple, Beech, Willow |

● Combination Remedies

Administer one Traumeel tablet directly into the mouth, three times per day, more often in acute situations. You may, alternatively, dissolve five tablets in water, and administer them over a one-day period. Reduce the medication as soon as you notice improvement. For dosages see the front inside cover.

When to Get Professional Help

Get a veterinarian's advice when you notice any eye injury, when you suspect a general infectious disease, or if the nictitating membrane remains apparent for an extended time.

What Are the Treatment Options?

The veterinarian is going to examine the external and internal parts of the eyes. Existing foreign particles must be removed under anesthesia. If your cat resists all external manipulations, the veterinarian will need to anesthetize the animal in order to be able to proceed effectively. Infectious diseases can be treated with homeopathic remedies by a veterinarian trained in health care techniques.

Prevention and Convalescent Care

Parasitic infestation is a common reason for the eversion of the third eyelid. You can avoid this problem by checking your cat's stool regularly. Whenever you treat the eyes of your cat topically, continue the treatment until the condition is completely healed. If you stop too early, the problem may start again, and may turn into a chronic inflammation.

Diseases of the External Ear

This problem is called otitis externa. It is a frequently encountered condition in cats, and can easily be recognized by the owner. It sometimes takes a long time for the ear to heal completely.

Symptoms

During the beginning phase of this condition the cat will hardly show any symptoms. It is only 1 to 2 weeks into the problem that you can expect to see signs, such as a tilted head or increased itching of one or both ears (one ear is usually more affected than the other). As scratching intensifies, moist wounds develop in and around the ear.

If you look inside the ear you will notice darkly discolored secretions in moist, caked, or encrusted form. At this point the ear is probably so painful, that any touch will be met with a discouraging hiss.

Causes

Ear mites are the culprits for this nasty problem. They deposit their excrement inside the ear, where it mixes with ear wax, leading to painful obstruction of the ear canal. Mites are transmitted between cats, as well as between cats and dogs, through close contact. If infected with mites by their mother, young kittens may react with severe illness.

Foreign objects, bacteria, and fungi can also cause otitis externa.

Self-Help

Important: Do not use Q-tips to clean the ears in the early stages of the disease, because you could aggravate the condition by pushing the secretions farther down into the passage.

Purchase a tool for ear cleaning in a veterinary office, or apply Peru balm (health food store), which will kill the mites. If the cat has created painful wounds by scratching around the ear, treat those areas with Calendula mother tincture, or apply Traumeel ointment for quick recovery.

● **Homeopathic Single Remedies**
Administer three to six times daily one oral dose of Calendula 6X.

Externally apply twice daily four to six drops of Calendula essence from the mother tincture. Gently massage the ear to distribute the medication. Continue for 3 to 7 days depending on the severity of the inflammation.

● **Bach Flowers**
Use Crab Apple for an otitis caused by mites, and add Cherry Plum if the cat suffers from painful itching ears.

● **Combination Remedies**
For inflammations the medication of choice is Mercurius-Heel. If your cat is in pain, or just sensitive to touch, add Traumeel tablets to the treatment. The dose for both medicines is one tablet three times daily.

When to Get Professional Help
In cases of stubborn ear problems you should have the cat treated by a veterinarian, in order to prevent the condition from becoming chronic.

What Are the Treatment Options?
The veterinarian uses an instrument, called an otoscope, to view and to assess the inflammation in the ear canal and the ear drum. This will allow a differentiation among mites, bacteria, or fungi as causative agents.

If the condition does not show signs of improvement, the practitioner will arrange for laboratory tests to determine which antibiotic, or other medication, is effective. In some cases injections may be necessary; in other cases ear drops will have to be administered for a certain time.

Prevention and Convalescent Care
The more frequently and thoroughly you examine your cat's ears, the less problems you will encounter, because you can stop an inflammation in the earliest stages. This advice is even more important for the care of nursing, or pregnant queens. Ear infections can be transmitted by the mother to the kittens, and the resulting ear infections are very serious (otitis interna, encephalitis, death).

Because of the mostly infectious nature of this problem, cats with otitis should be kept away from healthy cats, and their condition should be clearly established and treated. Inappropriate, or insufficiently long treatment of otitis results in severe chronic disease.

Ear Injuries

Symptoms
Your cat shows up with ears that are slit open and bloody.

Othematoma is a special lesion of the outer ear (the pinna). It consists of a broken blood vessel between the skin and the cartilage of the ear, which leads to an accumulation of blood and a resulting swelling that looks like a small pillow. The cat reacts to the imbalanced feeling in the ear by shaking its head, which makes the condition worse.

Ear injuries are most commonly the result of territorial fighting. The hematoma of the ear starts with an itching local inflammation, which drives the cat crazy in the urge to scratch and shaking of the head. While the scratching and shaking gives some relief, the ensuing internal damage of small blood vessels makes the condition worse.

Self-Help

An external injury should be treated with Calendula ointment. A swelling from a hematoma should be covered with a thin layer of Traumeel ointment. Both medications should be repeated three times daily. Apply the ointment gently and in a thin layer.

● Homeopathic Single Remedies

Arnica 12X is the choice for ear injuries. Treatment must be continued for 2 to 3 weeks because it takes many weeks for a hematoma to become fully resorbed.

● Bach Flowers

For deep and internal injuries administer Rescue Remedy, or Star of Bethlehem.

● Combination Remedies

Your cat may get better if you treat it with Traumeel tablets for 3 weeks. Dosages are listed on the inside front cover.

When to Get Professional Help

Serious ear injuries should be treated by a veterinarian.

What Are the Treatment Options?

You can manage most of the more common ear problems successfully at home. Othematoma, though, is frequently hard to clear up by yourself. Surgical correction is often necessary. Your veterinarian will advise you on the presurgical care and on the support of the cat following the operation.

Prevention and Convalescent Care

Ear injuries are most frequent in male outdoor cats, who are innate fighters. The best way to stop this behavior is by neutering the cat.

Inflammatory Lesions of the Mouth

Inflammation of the gums and of the mucosal lining of the mouth are called *gingivitis* and *stomatitis*. Older cats develop gingivitis quite frequently as a chronic condition. Left untreated, this problem can progress into stomatitis.

Symptoms

(A) *Gingivitis* is characterized by reddened, swollen, sometimes bleeding gum lines. Mucosal tissue may grow like polyps, and form pockets, which harbor bacterial growth. The longer the condition is allowed to proceed, the less chance the animal will be able to eat. Bloody saliva may be oozing from the mouth.

(B) *Stomatitis* may develop in localized areas of the mouth, forming small red spots, or tiny ulcerated pus containing patches. At this stage the general condition and behavior of the animal are uninhibited. However, if the stomatitis extends over the mucosa of the whole mouth, there is usually a generalized disease at the root of the problem. Symptoms like apathy, fever, vomiting, diarrhea, or pale mucosals frequently accompany this type of stomatitis.

Causes

(A) Tooth tartar (page 41) is the most common cause of gingivitis. Viral, bacterial, or fungal infections may also cause this problem.

(B) Localized inflammation could be attributed to injuries from objects such as needles, bone splinters, fish bones, or wood splinters. Severe cases of stomatitis are usually part of a systemic disease, such as viral infections (e.g., panleukopenia, leukemia, FRC, etc.).

Self-Help

For the treatment of the mouth you need to apply a rinse. Sage tea will work if you have a tolerant calm cat. Another alternative is a mixture of Arnica, Calendula, and Myrrh. Ask the pharmacist to mix it for you from the stock tinctures. Take one teaspoon of this mixture in one glass of warm water, and rinse the mouth several times.

● Homeopathic Single Remedies

Mercurius 12X is indicated for the treatment of highly offensive mouth odor.

Hepar sulfuris C30 should be given to cats whose gum lines show inflammation and pus, who are very sensitive to being touched around the head and face, and who seek warm places. Treat these patients for 4 days.

● Bach Flowers

Symptoms	Treatment
Tooth tartar	Crab Apple
Repeated gingivitis or stomatitis	Chestnut Bud
Apathy	Wild Rose
Inflammation after injury	Star of Bethlehem

● Combination Remedies

To treat a painful inflammation use Traumeel tablets, but for pus containing conditions you should administer Mercurius-Heel.

Dosages for all remedies are listed on the inside front cover.

When to Get Professional Help

Seek professional help if you notice heavy tartar deposits or if the cat shows symptoms of systemic disease.

What Are the Treatment Options?

(A) If tartar is the cause, it must be removed before anything else can be done. If the animal is not getting better, veterinary drugs should be considered.

(B) Heart and lung need to be evaluated thoroughly, and the mouth checked carefully. A blood test might also be needed if a viral infection is suspected.

For moderately ill cats there are drugs available that lower the fever, and that can be combined with the administration of Nosodes. Severely ill cats may need intravenous infusions and, in some cases, immune serum (page 121).

Prevention and Convalescent Care

If tartar is the cause, see page 41.

It is important to keep booster vaccinations current because viral infections like pneumonitis may cause oral diseases as described above.

Injuries of the Mouth

Young kittens are especially prone to head injuries. Extra caution can help avoid most of these cases.

Symptoms

The cat salivates, scratches its mouth and head frequently, and appears generally nervous. There may be blood-tinged saliva along the edges of the lips. Other indicators of head injuries are abnormal position of the jaws or swollen areas on the head.

Causes

Outdoor cats have a high number of injuries of the head because they get hit by cars. Typical occurrences are bruises, blunt impact trauma, and fractures of bones and teeth.

Jumping from lofty heights, like balconies, and trees, frequently causes sprains, contusions, and sometimes fractures of the lower jaw.

Kittens are often victims of their playfulness: needles, with and without threads, rubber bands, bone splinters, and many other objects can lead to injuries of the mouth. These injuries can be life threatening if not discovered in time.

Self-Help
Important: Accidents call for immediate emergency treatments to save lives. Take your cat to a practitioner's office without delay!

● **Homeopathic Single Remedies**
Arnica 12X should be given every 30 minutes for the first few hours following the injury.

● **Bach Flowers**

Symptoms	Treatment
Acute emergency or shock	Rescue Remedy
Physical injury	Star of Bethlehem

● **Combination Remedies**
Give your cat one Traumeel tablet every 1 to 2 hours until the condition is visibly improved.

Dosages for all remedies are listed on the inside front cover.

When to Get Professional Help
All accidents should be referred to a veterinary emergency clinic without delay!

What Are the Treatment Options?
A thorough examination will reveal the presence of any fractures or injuries that might require immediate surgical correction. Anesthesia would be necessary for operations to remove foreign objects or to fix a broken or dislocated jaw.

Prevention and Convalescent Care
Pay attention to loose objects lying around, especially needles.

Outdoor cats can only be protected from the risk of accidents by turning them into indoor cats. Remember that you need to keep a kitten inside from birth if you want to have a true indoor cat. If you want to allow your cat to be an outdoor cat, the animal should be spayed/neutered (page 19).

Tooth Tartar

Tartar, or plaque formation, appears as brown-gray discolored deposits along the teeth. There is usually heavier tartar deposit along the molars. If left unattended, the deposits can lead to severe and painful health problems. While Persian cats may show deposits relatively early in their lives, older cats are more likely to be affected.

Symptoms
Tooth tartar begins with thin deposits on the teeth, which are thickened and hardened by absorption of salts and minerals. They can cover the whole tooth, and lead to severe inflammation of the gum line. Bacteria will quickly settle in the deposits, causing more inflammation, ulceration, and bleeding.

Advanced ulcerated gingivitis causes the cat intolerable pain when the animal is trying to eat. Bad mouth odor, and salivation soon follow.

Causes
Inherited breed disposition, as well as generalized constitutional susceptibility, are mainly responsible for this problem.

Self-Help
If you catch the condition in its early stages, you can scrape off the deposits with your fingernail.

● **Homeopathic Single Remedies**

Borax 12X is the treatment of choice when you find your cat drooling suspiciously, or if you notice small blister-like inflammations around the teeth. A key symptom for Borax treatment is the fear of downward motion. For additional treatment suggestions see gingivitis on page 39.

If your cat shows a disposition for plaque formation, treat the animal with either Calcium carbonicum C30 or with Phosphorus C30 as a constitutional support (page 120). Give the medication once every 5 days to increase general resistance to disease.

● **Bach Flowers**

If your cat has a tendency to have tooth deposits, administer Crab Apple. If deposits have already formed and need to be removed, give the cat Gentian.

● **Combination Remedies**

Administer Traumeel and Mercurius-Heel.

For dosages see inside front cover.

When to Get Professional Help

Heavy dental plaque must be removed by a veterinarian.

What Are the Treatment Options?

Moderate dental plaque can be removed with a metal spoon scraper by a veterinarian trained in health care techniques. If, however, the cat resists the necessary restraint, or if the deposits are heavy, the veterinarian must clean the entire set of teeth under anesthesia with a specific ultrasonic instrument.

Prevention and Convalescent Care

Make sure that you offer your cat a well-balanced and varied diet (page 12). It is quite possible that cats, like humans, build up tartar if their nutrition lacks variety.

If your cat appears to be predisposed to plaque formation, try to get into the habit of cleaning the teeth with a cotton swab dipped in peroxide, or with a moist piece of cloth dipped in powdered chalk.

Inflammation of the Pharynx

The region of the pharynx is considered "defensive territory" because it harbors the tonsils and a variety of glands. An inflammation of this area is called pharyngitis. This condition may be localized, or may be part of a generalized disease. Tonsillitis may occur alone, or as part of a systemic disorder.

Symptoms

Inflammations of the pharynx appear as red mucosals with whitish deposits, or small pus-containing pustules. Swallowing becomes visibly impaired, and the glands in the area are soon included in the process.

Tonsillitis is mostly restricted to the tonsils. They appear enlarged, red, and irregular.

Causes

The majority of pharyngeal inflammations are caused by colds, drafts, wetness, as well as by changes in diet and by food that is served too cold. A variety of injuries in this area are not uncommon. Internal diseases, such as any one of the viral infections within FRC, may cause tonsillitis as secondary symptoms.

Self-Help

The application of a neck and throat compress, is easy and highly effective. Soak a towel in cold water into which you have mixed vinegar. Use three parts water with one part vinegar. See directions on page 45.

● Homeopathic Single Remedies
Aconitum C30 is indicated if the pharyngitis was caused by a cold draft or wind. Choose Belladonna C30 if there are symptoms such as fever, swollen glands, or sensitivity to touch.

● Bach Flowers
For an acute condition, use Centaury. However, use Larch if the animal appears weak and lethargic.

● Combination Remedies
Angina-Heel is indicated, at one tablet, three to six times daily. If you add Traumeel to this treatment by alternating between the two medications, the throat will heal much faster. In this case, give three tablets of each remedy per day.

Dosages for all remedies are listed on the inside front cover.

When to Get Professional Help
Seek the advice of a veterinarian if the condition does not show improvement, or if you suspect a viral infection.

What Are the Treatment Options?
Following a close exam of the throat region the veterinarian will select the medications that are most specific for the type of inflammation at hand.

If natural remedies do not have the desired effect the veterinarian will administer antibiotics. For this purpose it is necessary to take a culture from the pharyngeal mucosa.

Prevention and Convalescent Care
Cats who are sensitive to cold weather conditions should be kept inside. In addition, you should remember never to feed your cat cold, refrigerated foods. High-quality feline nutrition (page 12) and current vaccination boosters (page 17) strengthen the general immune system.

Diseases of the Respiratory and Circulatory Systems

The process of inhaling air provides the body with oxygen and with the nitrogen that is necessary to synthesize proteins. Air passes from the nasopharyngeal space through the bronchial ducts into the lungs. Here the oxygen enters the bloodstream, and the carbon dioxide is eliminated. The rhythm of the heart contractions moves the oxygenated blood through the arteries to all of the body's tissues. There, the cells deliver their carbon dioxide back into the blood, which carries it through the veins to the heart, and back to the lungs. With the next exhalation the carbon dioxide is eliminated.

Diseases of the respiratory system may affect any single organ or a group of organs. The latter is more common. Nasal catarrh is a relatively common problem in cats. In most cases it is a consequence of viral infections of the respiratory complex (page 90).

Circulatory diseases are relatively rare in cats. When they do occur, it is most frequently associated with old age. Heart problems in young cats are generally caused by congenital conditions.

Nose Bleeding

Symptoms
Blood is oozing out of one or both nostrils—either sporadically or continually. Both color and degree of blood flow are important indicators of their causes.

Causes
Most nose bleeding (epistaxis) is caused by accidents, such as falls from a window, car accidents, or foreign bodies like needles, splinters, and grains that get stuck in the nasal mucosa.

Infectious diseases and tumors can cause nasal deformations, which may lead to chronic nose bleeding.

Important: If the cat experiences repeated nose bleeds, and if you find it difficult to stop the bleeding, there is a possibility that liver disease or blood disorders are at the root of the problem.

Self-Help
Use Rescue cream externally to alleviate the condition, or place a cool compress on the nose.

● **Homeopathic Single Remedies**
As in the case of any accident, you should first administer Arnica 12X, about every 30 minutes (see page 109).

If the bleeding does not stop quickly, begin a treatment with Phosphorus 12X for 10 days. A constitutional phosphorus cat (page 115) should receive Phosphorus C30 four times on the first day, and once daily on the following 4 days, one dose each time. Bleeding from the left nostril, which is accompanied by pale mucosals, should be cured by a 2-week treatment with Ferrum 12X.

● **Bach Flowers**

Symptoms	Treatment
Nose injury	Star of Bethlehem
Bleeding is accompanied by distraught behavior	Agrimony
Nose bleed after accident	Elm

Important: Administer Rescue Remedy after any accident, and follow with a combination of Elm and Star of Bethlehem.

● **Combination Remedies**

Nose bleeds are best treated with either Cinnamomum-Homaccord or Phosphor-Homaccord. Administer the medication in the drinking water or right into the mouth via a disposable syringe. Phosphor is the choice for bleeding, nasal catarrh, and for pneumonia.

In acute situations you can give both medications every 30 minutes. Once the bleeding has stopped, continue for one more day.

Dosages for all remedies are listed on the inside front cover

When to Get Professional Help

Professional help is needed if there is a foreign body lodged inside the nasal passage, or if you cannot stop the bleeding. Most accidents should also be followed up with a professional exam.

What Are the Treatment Options?

First, the cause of the bleeding must be established. Anesthesia is necessary if a tumor or foreign body is suspected.

Prevention and Convalescent Care

Vaccinations (page 17) are the best prevention of nasal bleeding due to viral infections.

Laryngitis

The larynx is where sounds are formed. Laryngitis is present when your cat's meow sounds are distorted.

Symptoms

A hoarse meow and a cough are sure signs of laryngitis. The inflammation causes difficulties in swallowing, and fever. Slightest pressure on the larynx will cause the cat to cough, and any touch will elicit pain reactions.

Causes

Viruses that are part of the FRC (page 90) cause most of these cases. Noninfectious causes are irritating gases, frequent meowing, and the occasional foreign body.

Self-Help

A neck compress will lower the inflammation quickly. To prepare the compress, add ½ teaspoon fruit vinegar to 8 oz. (¼ L) moderately cool water. Use this to soak a piece of cloth or a handkerchief, wrap it around your cat's neck, and cover it with a wool shawl, or something similar. Leave this "bandage" on for about 2 hours. When you take it off, dry the moist hair thoroughly, and repeat the procedure 12 hours later.

● **Homeopathic Single Remedies**

Spongia 12X is the remedy of choice when the animal suffers from cough, hoarseness, and tenderness if touched. Administer this medication for 10 to 12 days.

Drosera 12X is indicated if the cat shows aggravated cough with gagging, suffocating episodes, and, generally, when a previously minor condition gets worse. You can administer this medication more frequently as the condition appears acute.

● **Bach Flowers**

Symptoms	Treatment
With a chronic cough	Crab Apple
With difficult swallowing	Elm, Mimulus
With fever	Holly

● **Combination Remedies**
Administer Husteel, and Grip-Heel, alternating every 2 hours in cases where fever weakens your cat. Reduce the treatment as soon as the cat gets better.

Dosages for all remedies are listed on the inside front cover.

When to Get Professional Help
Seek professional advice if the condition continues for an extended period.

Important: If your cat exhibits acute breathing difficulties, the infection may pass into the lungs, and you should not delay taking the animal to a veterinarian.

What Are the Treatment Options?
The veterinarian will examine the lungs and the bronchial system, and will determine whether a foreign body might be the cause. In cases where breathing is impaired, the veterinarian might need to prescribe drugs that can more quickly reduce severe swelling of the larynx.

Prevention and Convalescent Care
Regular vaccination boosters are the best prevention (page 17). In addition, give your cat only toys that cannot be swallowed. Watch out for strong scents or gases that might be inhaled by your cat, and that might cause irritation.

Bronchitis

It is only in rare cases (e.g., inhalation of a foreign body) that an inflammatory condition is restricted to the trachea. In most cases the bronchi and the trachea are affected simultaneously. This is called a tracheobronchitis.

Symptoms
The cat becomes lethargic, weak, and retreats into a quiet, dark corner. You can hear the animal cough, and the frequency of breathing is accelerated. Sounds from the chest signal an accumulation of mucus, which the animal is unable to expectorate. As the condition advances, the cat keeps its mouth open in order to be able to breathe, and exhaling becomes very painful.

Causes
Viral infections affect the mucosals severely, giving way to secondary bacterial infections and painful inflammation.

Self-Help
If you notice that the mucus can't be coughed up readily, it is best to prepare a chamomile inhalation, as described on page 102.

Important: This inflammation must be treated until it is completely gone in order to prevent permanent damage and to avoid a chronic condition.

2

● Homeopathic Single Remedies

If the cat's general well-being is not affected by the cough, you can use the same treatment as for laryngitis (page 45).

Ipecacuanha 6X is the right medication for a cough that is accompanied by vomiting but lacks any deposits on the tongue. Once the tracheitis spreads to the lungs, you need to proceed as described on pages 47–49.

● Bach Flowers

Symptoms	Treatment
Apathy, lack of responsiveness	Wild Rose
Lethargy, weakly motivated	Gorse
With productive cough	Crab Apple
Fever, severe coughing episodes	Holly

● Combination Remedies

All remedies that are listed for laryngitis are also suitable for tracheitis (page 45). Viropect powder is another effective treatment. You need to administer one pinch every 3 hours for 8 to 10 days by placing the powder directly into the mouth or into the drinking water.

Dosages for all remedies are listed on the inside front cover.

When to Get Professional Help

Get professional help if the treatment does not visibly improve the condition within 3 days or if you suspect pneumonia.

What Are the Treatment Options?

The most important part of a general exam will be listening to the lungs. This will determine a specific treatment mode.

If a viral infection is suspected, a serological test will diagnose the type of infection, and an antibiotic susceptibility test can be processed by a veterinarian (page 120).

Prevention and Convalescent Care

Cats that are susceptible to tracheobronchitis should be kept warm and treated protectively, especially during fall and winter.

Breed Dispositions

Because of their flattened head, Persian cats tend to suffer more from infections of the airways.

Pneumonia

Bronchitis can develop into pneumonia. When bronchi and lungs are affected simultaneously, it is called a bronchopneumonia.

Symptoms

The cat develops a high fever of 104°F (40°C) or more, it refuses food, and is lethargic. Coughing may be apparent, and breathing becomes labored to the point of breathing through the open mouth. Exhaling is especially painful at this stage. The animal wants to retreat and be left alone. Minor efforts, like picking the animal up and transporting it to the veterinary clinic, can lead to severe lack of oxygen, and circulatory complications.

Causes

A variety of negative factors may cause the body to lose some of its normal resistance, and make it susceptible to agents that, ultimately, cause the pneumonia. Such factors may be weather changes, stress, fights with other animals, dietary changes, or the addition of another pet competing for attention. Viruses, like herpes or Calici, may damage the cells to begin with, thus preparing the organism for further infections by bacteria, fungi, or parasites (e.g., roundworms).

Other infections, like feline leukemia and FIP, can, also weaken the immune system to the point of paving the way for pneumonia.

Self-Help

Important: Treatment of pneumonia must respond to your home treatment right away. If 6 to 12 hours elapse without any visible improvement, you must take your cat to a veterinary clinic for emergency treatment.

● Homeopathic Single Remedies
During the first few days administer alternating doses of Phosphorus 12X and Bryonia 6X every 2 hours. Once you notice improvement, reduce the doses slowly.

Important: This treatment should be continued for at least 8 to 10 days, or longer if necessary.

● Bach Flowers

Symptoms	Treatment
Apathy, lack of responsiveness	Wild Rose
Distraught, lack of reaction and attention	Clematis
Changes of diet or weather	Walnut
Pain and severe inflammation	Holly
Loss of resistance, weakness	Centaury

● Combination Remedies
The most important medication for the treatment of pneumonia is Bryaconeel, which you dissolve in water and administer three to six times daily, one tablet each. You may want to treat your cat every 30 minutes in the beginning stages of the illness. Gripp-Heel or Phosphor-Homaccord are equally effective. The first is dosed at one tablet, three to fivr times daily, the latter at five drops, three to six times daily.

Dosages for all remedies are listed on the inside front cover.

When to Get Professional Help
Take your cat to a veterinarian as soon as you observe severe general symptoms, like difficulties in breathing. Also, seek help when your treatment has not shown prompt signs of improvement.

What Are the Treatment Options?
The mouth, throat, and lungs will be examined. An x-ray may be required. Blood cultures and antibiotic sensitivity tests may also be necessary to define a diagnosis. Certain conditions may require treatment with antibiotics and/or drugs that reduce the mucus formation in order to initiate healing.

Prevention and Convalescent Care
The most reliable prevention is based on keeping vaccination boosters current (page 17) and providing highly nutritious meals (page 12), combined with regular maintenance schedules.

Once you have a cat that is ill with pneumonia, keep it away from other animals and provide it with a warm, and quiet bed. While food intake is not important during the first 2 days of illness, you must make sure that your cat takes in enough fluid to make up for the dehydration due to fever and mucus production. If the animal is not drinking water, you can dissolve the homeopathic medicine in water, or in tea, and instill it via a disposable syringe (without needle!) right into the mouth (directions on page 103).

For how to feed sick cats, see page 106.

If the cat is treated by a veterinarian, directions for home care will be given to you at that time.

Breed Dispositions

The flattened shape of a Persian's head predisposes it to respiratory tract ailments.

Anemia

Anemia is a condition, which is characterized by lowered numbers of red blood cells and by a reduction in hemoglobin. The result of anemia is a lack of oxygen and nutrients in the body's tissues.

Symptoms

The color of the cat's skin, particularly at the nose and ears, is pale, and the mucosals around the eyes and mouth are white or transparent like porcelain. The animal appears weak, lethargic, and refuses to eat. Breathing and pulse are accelerated, and, in advanced stages, lack of oxygen may lead to shortness of breath and heart problems.

Causes

Shock and resulting anemia may be initiated by extensive injuries, like those caused by cars or by agricultural equipment.

Among the viral infections, anemia is most frequently caused by feline leukemia, pneumonitis, and FIP.

Parasites, such as ticks, or intestinal infestation with tapeworms, can also cause anemic conditions.

In addition, there are parasites, called Hemobartonella, which directly invade and destroy the red blood cells.

If there are bone marrow problems in any way, anemia may develop. A lack of nutritional iron can also cause anemia.

Self-Help

After an accident, the cat should be taken to an emergency clinic in order to provide life-saving medical first aid. How to provide other support is discussed on page 108.

● Homeopathic Single Remedies

Arnica 12X should be given after any accident (see page 109). For severe bleeding, add Phosphorus 12X to the initial treatment.

When dealing with an anemic cat, who is also dehydrated and does not tolerate being handled, administer five globules of China 6X three times daily until the animal has recovered its vitality.

● Bach Flowers

Symptoms	Treatment
Problems arising from an accident	1. Rescue Remedy 2. Star of Bethlehem, Elm
Worm infestation	Crab Apple
Lethargy, tiredness	Olive

● Combination Remedies

Traumeel is used for injuries. For infected wounds, Arnica-Heel will provide pain relief. If the cat appears weak and exhausted, give it China-Homaccord, until it has regained its strength. If lack of iron is the cause of the anemia, give Ferrum-Homaccord, five drops, three times daily.

Crataegus-Heel is a medication which is used to treat anemic cats whose cardiovascular system is affected by this blood disorder.

Dosages for all remedies are listed on the inside front cover.

When to Get Professional Help

If you do not know what caused the anemia, or whether or not you are dealing with an anemic animal, get professional help.

What Are the Treatment Options?

A blood analysis will establish the type and degree of disease. Parasitism will, also, be ruled out, or treated if present.

Severely anemic patients may require a blood transfusion, which would also contain iron supplements.

Antibiotics may be needed if the condition is caused by infectious agents. If, however, the anemia is caused by FIP or feline leukemia, the chance for recovery is quite poor.

Prevention and Convalescent Care

Regular vaccination boosters against leukemia and FIP (page 93) are needed for all cats, in order to prevent disease and to prevent contracting disease from other cats.

Keeping your cat worm-free (page 16) makes the animal resistant to diseases.

If you live in a rural area, try to keep your cat close to home during the peak harvesting activities, because major injuries occur specifically at this time. Animals that are hit by cars or large equipment experience extensive lesions and severe blood loss.

Diseases of the Digestive Tract

Cats have a digestive tract that is typical for carnivorous animals: There is an almost square mouth cavity, and 30 teeth, including the significant canine teeth for tearing meat. A single stomach cavity follows, which is responsible for the predigestion of proteins. The small intestine is where proteins, carbohydrates, and fats are broken down, and absorbed together with vitamins, minerals, and trace elements. All digestive processes are supported though liver and pancreas functions; both organs contribute directly to the intestines via a duct system. The pancreas produces important digestive enzymes. For pancreatic diseases see page 76. The large intestine is approx. 8 in. (20 cm) long, and it delivers water to the body's organ systems.

Diseases of the digestive tract may or may not affect the general well-being of the animal. The majority of the symptoms consist of lack of appetite, constipation, vomiting, or diarrhea.

Hair Balls (Bezoares)

Cats accumulate hair in their digestive tract because the fur sticks to their rough tongue during the grooming process, and is swallowed. Under normal conditions, the hair is discharged with the stool. However, hair may accumulate and form hair balls, called bezoares, when there is an abnormal amount of hair, like during the shedding season, when a cat suffers from hair loss, or in long-haired cats, which are not brushed regularly. The resulting problems vary in the degree of severity.

Symptoms

During the shedding season cats vomit hair balls more frequently. There may be clumps of hair, food particles, and mucus apparent in the vomited matter. Hair balls may cause an inflammation of the stomach lining if they remain in the stomach, where they irritate the mucosa. Gastritis will become apparent when the cat starts to gag and vomit, and then is lethargic.

It is only in very rare instances that hair balls lead to occlusion of the stomach or intestine. The latter would find your cat in a generally weak condition, highly sensitive to touch, and with a distended, painful belly.

Causes

Hair balls aggregate in the stomach because of the continuous movement, which causes clumping of food, fluids, and hairs. If the clumps are not moved along in the digestive tract, they can get bigger, and can cause problems.

Self-Help

Hair ball blockages are easily resolved with vegetable oils or with the oil from a can of sardines. Kittens receive 1 teaspoon, and cats get 2 teaspoons per treatment.

Important: If the cat shows signs of pain, and if you suspect a hair ball blockage, take your cat to a veterinarian immediately. This condition could be life-threatening.

● **Homeopathic Single Remedies**

Opium 30C will relieve an aching belly. Give your cat ten globules, dissolved in water. Repeat this in short intervals.

During the shedding season, you can give your cat five globules of Sulfur 30C to improve the condition of the hair coat.

● **Bach Flowers**

Symptoms	Treatment
Apathy, lethargy	Wild Rose
Severe exhaustion	Olive
To stimulate excretion	Crab Apple

● **Combination Remedies**

For the treatment of gastritis, use Gastricumeel; Nux vomica should be used for painful digestive conditions.

Dosages for all remedies inside front cover.

When to Get Professional Help

If your cat continues to vomit, and if you notice symptoms like fever, apathy, or pain, do not hesitate to seek professional advice.

What Are the Treatment Options?

The practitioner will try to eliminate the hair balls by administering calming and antispastic natural medications. If all natural, conservative methods fail to eliminate the bezoares, surgical removal may be necessary.

Prevention and Convalescent Care

Regular, thorough hair care (page 104) is essential, especially during the shedding season.

If hair is falling out because of underlying diseases, such as skin conditions or parasitism, the disease must be treated to remove the source of the problem.

Your cat will appreciate it if you always provide a potted plant of wheatgrass or oats. This will help regulate its digestive functions.

Vomiting

Vomiting is an accompanying symptom of many disorders. It is a process that is stimulated by adverse reactions in the gastrointestinal tract, which, in turn, activate the specific nerve center for vomiting in the medulla oblongata, an extension of the spinal cord.

Cats vomit under normal conditions for the purpose of purging indigestible plant materials or hair balls from their digestive tract. There is nothing to worry about when this occurs. If, however, a cat vomits repeatedly in a short interval, if the vomiting is accompanied by diarrhea, shows blood tinged materials, or leads to general signs of disease, the animal should be examined by a health care practitioner.

Symptoms

The cat starts to choke and cough, which results in vomiting, whereby undigested stomach contents are expelled. In order to identify the cause of the trouble, it is important to observe the color and consistency of the vomited material. Appearance ranges from mucoid-foamy to yellowish-stringy, or blood-tinged. Also, pay attention to the time when vomiting occurs, e.g., before or after a meal. All descriptive observations are important for the veterinarian's diagnosis.

Important: If you notice blood in the vomited material take your cat to a veterinarian immediately.

Causes

There are many causes for vomiting: Hair balls, and foreign objects in the stomach, gastric inflammation or ulcers, or parasites. Cats may also vomit if their food upsets their digestive system.

Other causes include viral, bacterial, and fungal infections, as well as poisons, allergies, and other irritations. As an accompanying symptom, vomiting is seen in general diseases caused by disorders of the liver, gallbladder, pancreas, kidney, or of the digestive tract.

Self-Help

● Homeopathic Single Remedies

If kittens vomit approximately 10 minutes after a meal consisting of milk, the milk might have gone bad. In that case, treat them for 3 to 5 days, several times daily with Aethusa 6X giving each kitten three to five globules per dose.

Vomiting accompanied by coughing, without deposits on the tongue, should be treated with Ipecacuanha 6C.

Nux vomica 12X is needed when vomiting is complicated by constipation.

Pulsatilla 12X is preferred if you notice a lack of thirst and significant changes of behavior. Or, you can alternate the two latter medications, especially if you are unsure of the cause of the trouble.

● Bach Flowers

Symptoms	Treatment
Changing stool consistency, constipation	Scleranthus
Apathy	Wild Rose
As cleanser for over-burdened organism	Crab Apple

● Combination Remedies

Give your cat Nux vomica-Homaccord three to six times daily, directly into the mouth or in the drinking water.

Dosages for all remedies are listed on the inside front cover.

When to Get Professional Help

Get advice from a veterinarian if pet vomits more than four times in one day, of if vomiting episodes continue over several days, or if the animal appears generally ill. Take the animal to the veterinarian immediately if you suspect poisoning or viral infections.

What Are the Treatment Options?

The practitioner will, most likely, analyze stool and blood samples to determine specific remedies. In some cases, x-rays of the abdominal area are necessary, or the digestive tract may have to be examined with a special scope that is passed through the pharynx into the stomach.

Prevention and Convalescent Care

If hair balls are the cause of the vomiting, see page 51; for viral infections, see pages 90–94, and for nutritional problems, see page 12.

Diarrhea

Diarrhea is the result of gastroenteritis, which may be part of a number of general diseases. It is also a reaction by the body to rid itself of potentially toxic substances.

Toxins, viruses, and parasites cause intestinal inflammation, which leads to inadequate water resorption in the large intestine, and produces soft to fluid stools. Because both stomach and intestines are affected simultaneously in the majority of cases, the condition is generally referred to as gastroenteritis.

Symptoms

The first sign of diarrhea is often a soiled anal area. The cat intensifies its grooming efforts, and seeks the litterbox frequently. If the diarrhea continues, fever and other generalized symptoms will most likely develop, as well as weakness, apathy, and weight loss. Left untreated, the condition worsens, minerals are lost with the fluids, and severe organic damage may occur.

For the selection of the right treatment it is important that you know the consistency of the stool, e.g., watery-thin, thick or frothy, does the stool shoot vigorously from the rectum, or does it take much urging, and pressing?

The color of the stool is equally important to locate the original problem. Liver (page 57) and pancreas (page 76) are usually at fault when the stool is white. If you notice light-colored blood in the stool it indicates a rectal disorder. Signs of dark or black blood originate most commonly in the small intestine.

Important: The advice of a veterinarian is essential in cases where you observe blood in the stool, especially if the condition persists longer than 2 days, and if the general well-being is visibly affected.

Causes

Diarrhea is often a secondary symptom of a primary disease like viral infections (e.g., FIP), bacterial infections (Coli, Salmonella), or disorders caused by protozoa and fungi.

Noninfectious causes are usually poor nutrition, parasites, poisoning, or allergic reactions, as well as tumors and foreign bodies.

Diarrhea may also accompany diseases of the liver, and of the pancreas, like diabetes, or it may be due to a hyperactive thyroid.

Self-Help

Place the cat on a two-day fast. Fluid should be offered in the form of herbal tea, e.g., chamomile, fennel, or black tea. A tea from the bark of oak trees disinfects and also has a calming effect on the intestine. Supplemental electrolytes (page 106) will protect the cat from dehydration.

● Homeopathic Single Remedies

Arsenicum album 12X is indicated if the diarrhea was caused by spoiled meats, if the stool flows mainly at night, and if the cat takes in very little fluids.

Pulsatilla 12X is the right treatment when the color and consistency of the stool change frequently, and the cat does not appear to be thirsty.

Use Podophyllum 6X in cases where the stool is yellow-brown, and it is eliminated under strong pressure.

● Bach Flowers

Symptoms	Treatment
Dehydration with vomiting, diarrhea	Rock Rose
Exhaustion	Olive
Severe loss of vitality	Wild Rose
To induce a cleansing process	Crab Apple

● Combination Remedies

Give your cat one tablet Diarrheel three to six times daily. Either grind it up or dissolve it in water, and give it directly into the mouth.

3

Another choice is Dysenteral, five drops, twice daily, for 4 days.

Dosages for all remedies are listed on the inside front cover.

When to Get Professional Help

Get help from a practitioner if the diarrhea persists after two days, and if general symptoms of disease appear.

Important: Take the cat to a veterinarian immediately if the skin elasticity shows obvious signs of dehydration. You can check for this by pulling up a skin fold at the side of the neck, and if it does not retract immediately then dehydration has set in.

What Are the Treatment Options?

Stool and blood analyses will determine the cause of the diarrhea. A severely dehydrated animal will receive an intravenous electrolyte infusion to fend off overacidification of the body and to replace lost minerals. In addition to herbal treatments, it may be necessary to administer antibiotics in order to kill bacterial colonies.

Nosodes should be considered if the condition appears to resist treatments.

Prevention and Convalescent Care

The right intestinal conditions prevail when you provide optimal nutrition (page 12). Do not offer foods which are either spoiled or indigestible, e.g., milk that is too cold or too hot.

After 2 days of fasting place your cat on a special enteric diet (page 106).

Regular vaccinations help prevent viral infections.

Watch out for ecto- and endoparasites (see pages 84–89).

Make sure that all poisonous plants, chemical cleansers, and detergents are stored out of reach of your cat.

Constipation

Constipation exists when fecal matter accumulates in the large intestine (colon) and transport movement stops. Since the large intestine is also the place for water resorption, the material dries out further, causing the rectum to expand.

The majority of cats who suffer from constipation are old, neutered, or long-haired.

Symptoms

The cat does not eliminate any or only very little stool. The animal turns lethargic, lies about inactively, and attempts repeatedly to void stool by straining in the litterbox. Check the litter to determine whether it is urine or stool that is being retained. As the condition progresses, the cat becomes more lethargic, the eyes appear sunken, and the body temperature remains low. The belly becomes visibly distended and hard. The cat feels pain if you try to lift it by the belly.

Causes

Most cases of constipation are caused by hair balls (page 51). Constipation can also be caused by the following: wrong nutrition, age-related intestinal sluggishness, swallowed foreign bodies, parasites, infectious diseases (page 90), and tumors of the ovaries or elsewhere in the abdominal cavity.

Important: A special form of constipation is caused by *intestinal occlusion* (ileus). This is mostly caused by lodged foreign bodies, torsion, or intestinal inversions. If a cat vomits frequently without eliminating any stool an ileus could be the cause. This is a life-threatening condition that must be attended to by a veterinarian immediately. If you have Opium 30C in the house administer it right away.

Self-Help

It only takes a tablespoon of oil from a can of sardines, or of paraffin oil to get a constipated intestine moving again. Raw liver is helpful too.

If the constipation is more stubborn you should use a warm, soapy water enema to be safe. Avoid all commercial human preparations to soften the stool.

● **Homeopathic Single Remedies**

Calcium carbonicum 12X will solve the problem if the cat is slow and gentle by nature.

Use Graphites 12X for cats who are lazy, eat a lot, and who suffer from skin rashes and brittle nails. One dose three times daily will lead to quick relief.

Nux vomica 12X is for the feline patient with spastic straining and a very tense back.

● **Bach Flowers**

Symptoms	Treatment
Sluggish intestine	Chicory, Elm
Intestinal cramping	Agrimony
Inhibited internal cleansing	Crab Apple
Tension	Oak

● **Combination Remedies**

Give a chronically constipated cat one tablet of Heelax after every meal. If metabolic disorders exist in the digestive system you should treat the animal with Nux vomica Homaccord. The latter treatments may also be combined.

For all dosages of all remedies see inside front cover.

When to Get Professional Help

Get professional help if your treatments are unsuccessful or if the cat shows general symptoms of disease.

What Are the Treatment Options?

The veterinarian will attempt to loosen the stool with the help of an enema, biological remedies, manual massage, as well as with fluid instillation. If nothing works, the abdomen must be opened under anesthesia, and the intestine emptied surgically.

Prevention and Convalescent Care

Create as much exercise opportunities as possible for your cat. A sluggish intestine is best stimulated by a diet that is varied and has optimal nutrient content (page 12). You can also enrich the food with bulk such as linseed, wheatgerm, oats, and vegetables (carrots). Specific enteric diets (pages 106–107) that are designed for weight reduction are also suitable for this condition. If the constipation is due to hair balls, see page 51; if worms are involved, see pages 87–89. Keep up worm treatments. If the problem was treated surgically follow the instructions of the veterinarian with respect to after-care and diet.

Breed Disposition

Longhaired cats, like Persians, suffer more often from hair balls than other breeds.

Diseases of the Liver

The liver participates in a large number of the body's metabolic functions. It is often compared to a chemical factory. The liver assists in the metabolism of proteins, carbohydrates, and fats. Other tasks include detoxification, breakdown and preparation of hormones, and regulation of the vitamin stores. Liver cells are very active, and allow signs of disease to surface only in the late stages of a problem. An inflammation of the liver (hepatitis) may be either *acute* or *chronic*. Acute hepatitis may be treatable, whereas the chronic form usually progresses to an irreversible cirrhosis.

Symptoms

Liver disease may be signaled by a variety of symptoms such as loss of appetite, salivation, repetitive diarrhea, or vomiting (bile).

If detoxification is incomplete, and toxins reach the brain, there may be symptoms of brain disorders, even coma. If the disease progresses, the gallbladder no longer processes the breakdown products of the red blood cells, which may lead to jaundice. At this stage the skin and mucosal surfaces appear light yellow.

Liver disease is also characterized by a darkly discolored urine, and by a light, clay-colored stool.

Causes

Infectious hepatitis can be caused by viruses, bacteria, fungi, parasites, or monocellular organisms.

Noninfectious hepatitis may be caused by poisoning, tumors, and by fatty degeneration.

Self-Help

Important: Whenever you suspect liver disease you should consult a veterinarian.

● Homeopathic Single Remedies

Natrium sulfuricum 12X, administered for 3 weeks, is the main choice of treatment for liver disease that is characterized by jaundice, vomiting of bile, bloating, pain in the area of the liver, and by profuse amounts of stool.

Lycopodium 12X should be administered for 2 to 3 weeks if the symptoms are a distended belly, flatulence, shiny dry stool, and if the condition gets worse between 4 P.M. and 8 P.M. in the evening.

● Bach Flowers

Symptoms	Treatment
Poor digestion	Gentian
Exhaustion	Olive
Fearful and mistrusting	Willow

● Combination Remedy

Hepeel is the most important remedy for liver disorders.

Another alternative is the alternating administration of Nux vomica Homaccord and Chelidonium Homaccord. The first is effective in cases of functional disorders of the liver and the digestive tract; the other is formulated for liver and gallbladder disorders. Administer five drops of each medication three times daily.

Dosages for all remedies are listed on the inside front cover.

When to Get Professional Help

If your cat shows any signs of jaundice or of liver disease, you should seek veterinary help immediately.

3

What Are the Treatment Options?

The stage of liver disease can be diagnosed with a blood analysis or with a liver biopsy. If advanced disease is present, the animal may need to be hospitalized for infusion treatments.

Prevention and Convalescent Care

The liver will greatly benefit from an optimal diet (page 12), because it is the central metabolic organ.

If your animal appears sick and has no appetite, offer only water for 2 days. Then, begin a liver diet. You can either cook the liver yourself, or you can buy a commercially available liver diet from your veterinarian.

Overweight cats should be placed on a weight-loss diet, and the bulk in their food should be increased.

Vaccinations are the pillars of preventive care (page 17).

Diseases of the Urinary Tract and Reproductive Organs

The kidneys produce urine. They are the central organs of the urinary tract. They purge the blood of substances that must be eliminated, participate in the water and electrolyte metabolism, and manufacture important vitamins and hormones. Other organs are the ureter, the bladder, and the urethra, which eliminates the urine.

An inflammation of the kidneys may be acute, or it may develop into a chronic form, resulting in kidney failure. Diseases of the kidneys mainly affect older cats. The urinary bladder, however, is not infrequently the site of disease. This is mostly due either to an inherited weakness or to poor maintenance and diet.

The reproductive organ system consists of the testes or ovaries (which harbor the germ cells), and of the spermatic duct or the oviduct. In the female cat the two oviducts join in the ovary. The short, but wide urethra ends in the vulva. In the tomcat the long spermatic ducts end in the narrow urethra, which is the site of frequent troubles.

Diseases of the male reproductive organs may be caused by malformations, or disorders of the testis, spermatic ducts, or penis. These disorders are especially important in breed stock.

Female reproductive organ disorders may be located anywhere, but most problems affect the uterus. This organ is particularly sensitive around the time of birth.

Acute Nephritis

This problem is rare in cats. If suspected, it must be treated quickly and specifically.

The cat expells less urine, the urine may be blood-tinged, the animal shows no sign of thirst, and the mouth has a sweet odor. The animal arches its back, and, with a painful stiff gait, returns frequently to the litterbox to urinate.

Other unspecific general symptoms of disease may appear, such as lethargy, weakness, dull fur, as well as lack of appetite, vomiting, or diarrhea.

Important: Your detailed observations are of great importance for the veterinarian. A good report of symptoms can save a life in cases of poisonings.

Causes
The cause may be an infection of the kidneys. Kidneys may also be damaged by urine retention that is caused by kidney stones or by poisoning with antifreeze or heavy metals, as well as by injuries from accidents, by medications that are toxic for the kidneys, or by severe blood loss.

Self-Help
Important: If you suspect kidney disease get professional help immediately. Use home remedies only as a first aid measure.

4

Make a sick bed for the cat in a warm and quiet area. Cover the cat to keep it warm.

● **Homeopathic Single Remedies**
If the kidney trouble was caused by an accident give the cat Arnica 12X (page 109).

Apis 12X is indicated when urine is retained, the cat won't drink, and when the animal does not like to be kept warm. Give the cat five globules three or more times daily until the urine is voided freely.

Belladonna 4X at one dose every 1 to 2 hours is indicated in cases of sudden onset of disease if the pupils are dilated and the urine is tinged red.

● **Bach Flowers**

Symptoms	Treatment
Urine retention due to stones	Rescue Remedy
To expel stones during obstruction	Crab Apple
Restless and painful cramping	Agrimony
Inflammation	Holly, Rock Rose

● **Combination Remedies**
Berberis-Homaccord is helpful in cases of painful cramping. Traumeel tablets are indicated for injuries and contusions. Use Apis-Homaccord for urine retention and edema. Albumoheel tablets should be used if albumin was found in the urine analysis and also for acute or chronic kidney disease. These medications may be given singly or combined.

For dosages of all remedies see inside front cover.

When to Get Professional Help
If you suspect kidney disease the cat should be examined by a veterinarian as soon as possible because kidney failure may be a life-threatening condition.

What Are the Treatment Options?
In order to determine the diagnosis and the treatment method the veterinarian will palpate the abdomen of the cat, and a blood analysis will establish values for kidney chemistries, which are indicative of specific diseases. An electrolyte infusion may be needed to replenish the cat's body fluids and to get the kidneys working again. A number of natural remedies are effective in unburdening the kidney functions in order to prevent uremia (urine poisoning of the blood).

If the kidney problem was caused by poisoning, the correct counteracting medication has to be found to heal the damage.

Prevention and Convalescent Care
Make sure that poisonous plants, medicines, and household cleaners are out of reach of the cat. Kittens particularly are in danger because of their playfulness and curiosity.

If your cat is recovering from a kidney disease you should feed a kidney diet with reduced protein content (page 107).

Chronic Nephritis

Chronic nephritis is the most frequently encountered form in cats. It occurs mainly in cats that are older than 10 years.

Symptoms
The fur appears dull and rough, often with dander, or with visible parasites. The nutritional condition is usually poor, the skin is dehydrated, and the cat has little or varying degrees of appetite. Vomiting and diarrhea are often present. The eyes appear dull, the mucosals are the color of porcelain, and

the oral mucosa is typically inflamed. The mouth emits a distinctly sweet odor.

The cat drinks more water because the kidney disorder has caused a loss of body fluids, particularly electrolytes. More urine is voided, its color is light, and it has hardly an odor. If the disease progresses, the cat can no longer eliminate all the substances that should be leaving the body through the urine. This condition may lead to uremia, which could be fatal.

Causes

Chronic nephritis may be the sequel to an acute inflammatory condition. However, the problem may also develop following some other longstanding disorder, like a chronic inflammation of the mouth, or it could be part of a generalized viral infection.

Self-Help

Important: Natural remedies should be used for kidney disorders *only* under the direct guidance of a veterinarian trained in heath care techniques.

● Homeopathic Single Remedies

Arsenicum album 30C, given for 8 days, is the right treatment for cats that are dehydrated, emaciated, with scaly skin, who are very thirsty, seek warmth, and whose condition is worse after midnight.

Mercurius 30C, also administered for 8 days, is indicated if there is frequent urge to urinate but voiding is sparse, and if the urine is cloudy and blood-tinged. The cat has a very offensive mouth odor, salivates during the night, and its tongue appears swollen, showing imprints of the teeth.

● Bach Flowers

Symptoms	Treatment
To aid recovery from chronic condition	Chestnut Bud
To cleanse after a poisoning	Crab Apple
Severe tiredness and exhaustion	Olive

● Combination Remedies

If the cat is suffering from an acute condition administer daily one ampule of Cantharis comp. S in the drinking water. Continue with one ampule, three times each week. Solidago comp. S may be used in the same manner for acute or chronic kidney and other urinary tract problems.

For dosages of all remedies see inside front cover.

When to Get Professional Help

A cat with chronic kidney problems should be seen by a veterinarian as soon as possible.

Important: If you suspect a kidney disorder try to collect a urine sample before you see the veterinarian.

What Are the Treatment Options?

Following a general examination the veterinarian will palpate the kidney area and then proceed to process blood and urine analyses. These will determine the diagnosis and therapeutic choices.

If the kidneys are severely damaged, the first action will be to give the cat intravenous infusions with electrolytes and glucose to stimulate healing.

If, however, the cause of the diseases is a primary leukemia, you should consider euthanasia (page 120) at this time, because the condition is not curable.

4

Prevention and Convalescent Care

Regular vaccinations are the best prevention against viral diseases (page 17). In addition, optimal nutrition (page 12) is the foundation for warding off disease.

If there are any signs of kidney disorders you should start your cat immediately on a kidney diet (page 107) with lowered protein content. You can either prepare the diet at home, or you can use the commercially available diets, which are easier to handle and store and which are carefully formulated to meet the needs of your cat.

Important: Make sure that you provide your cat with daily fresh drinking water in clean water bowls.

Cystitis

Cats suffer only rarely from cystitis.

Symptoms

An affected cat can be observed trying to urinate frequently. There are only dribbles, and the color may be tinged with blood. In other cases, the cat may be unable to hold the flow of urine, and bloody drops are left all over the house. There is obvious pain associated when touching the cat's abdomen and when the animal is straining to urinate.

The general condition is usually not affected. Fever is rare, but may occur due to bacterial infections.

Causes

Most cystitis cases are caused by urinary sediment or by calculi, which continue to irritate the mucosal lining of the bladder.

A cystitis may develop after a cat gets cold and wet during the fall season. Another cause of cystitis may be an ascending infection, which started in the urethra. This is mostly a problem in female cats because they have very short urethras.

Self-Help

Important: Cystitis must be treated specifically and quickly in order to prevent the development of chronic conditions.

● Homeopathic Single Remedies

Belladonna 6X, given every 2 hours, is indicated in acute cases where urine retention, blood in the urine, and dribbling are symptomatic.

Cantharis 6X is the treatment of choice when a painful urge to urinate are predominant, and when bloody urine is voided drop by drop. Start with treatments every 2 hours, and reduce to daily doses once improvement has begun.

● Bach Flowers

Symptoms	Treatment
Restlessness	Agrimony
Sudden onset of disease	Elm
Urge with urine retention	Cherry Plum
Severe cystitis pain	Holly

● Combination Remedies

Treat cystitis with Reneel tablets. In addition, you can use Berberis-Homaccord for inflammatory conditions with cramping, or Plantago-Homaccord for bladder irritation and urging.

Dosages for all remedies are listed on the inside front cover.

When to Get Professional Help

A cat with cystitis should be seen by a professional in order to avoid the development of chronic disease.

What Are the Treatment Options?
Important: If you suspect a cystitis, try to get a urine specimen before you see the veterinarian.

First, a diagnosis must be determined by palpating the abdomen, which is in most cases very tense. In addition, an x-ray or an ultrasound exam may be necessary. If the bladder is full, a catheter will be inserted to relieve the pressure. The urine may be cultured to determine whether a bacterial infection is involved. A veterinarian may need to administer medication to reduce the cramping and an antibiotic to kill bacterial infections.

Prevention and Convalescent Care
Cats who have an established disposition for cystitis should be especially guarded during the wet and cold seasons. Warmth, fresh water, and bladder teas support healthy kidney functions.

If your cat tends to get cystitis repeatedly, you should initiate a full-length intensive bladder treatment regimen in order to prevent any potential ascending kidney problems.

Urinary Stones

The formation of urinary sediment and stones (urolithiasis) are encouraged by exclusive feeding of dry foods, by lack of fresh water consumption, lack of exercise, and by castration. Tomcats are predisposed because their relatively long narrow urethra may be irritated by minor accumulations of sediment. The female cat's wide and short urethra passes even larger calculi more easily.

Symptoms
The first signs of urinary deposits are sediments,

blood, and pus. If the sediment irritates the urethra, there will soon be signs of serious difficulties in urination, at times yielding only drops.

The cat is meowing in pain because of the burning sensation during urination. If a stone is blocking the urethra the urine may be backed up all the way to the kidney. At this stage the cat is at risk of a bladder rupture and of uremia.

Causes
Bladder stones are mainly caused by wrong maintenance, wrong nutrition, high magnesium in the diet, or by inflammatory disorders. A hereditary disposition may also contribute to the problem.

Self-Help
● **Homeopathic Single Remedies**
Lycopodium 30C is indicated when the cat retains urine, when severe repeated pressing yields only partial elimination, and when red sediment is visible in the urine. Use this medication also when metabolic disorders exist, and when the liver is involved in the disease.

Administer Berberis 12X for 2 to 3 weeks when the cat experiences frequent, painfully burning urination, and when the urine is foamy, with reddish-tinged sediment.

● **Bach Flowers**

Symptoms	Treatment
Great difficulties and pain	Rescue Remedy
Restlessness and pain	Agrimony
Inability to expel calculi	Crab Apple

● **Combination Remedies**
Berberis-Homaccord is the most important treatment, especially in cases of repetitive urging.

Dosages for all remedies are listed on the inside front cover.

When to Get Professional Help

Seek professional help if your cat shows signs of pain when urine is being retained or if your pet appears lethargic.

What Are the Treatment Options?

If the urethra is obstructed by sediment or calculi, it will be necessary to anesthetize the cat and to flush the urinary tract. Large bladder stones can only be removed surgically. If a chronic cystitis appears to cause the sediment formation the practitioner would most likely treat the inflammatory disorder first.

Prevention and Convalescent Care

Pay close attention to the amount of exercise your cat receives, to regular meal times, and to optimal diet composition (pages 12 to 15). Should your cat be disposed to urinary sediment formation you should feed the animal a specific low magnesium diet (no more than 20 mg/100 kcal; (see page 12).

Because alkaline urine encourages the formation of bladder stones it is possible to add 0.8 g of ammonium chloride to the food in order to acidify the urine.

Important: The formation of urinary calculi is a constitutional problem, which should be dealt with by regular urine analysis.

Breed Dispositions

Persian cats are predisposed to form urinary calculi.

Diseases of the Uterus

Symptoms

(A) Inflammation of the uterus. One to three days after delivering, the queen develops a fever, becomes lethargic, and loses interest in her offspring. In severe cases the cat may vomit, get diarrhea, become exhausted, and get severely dehydrated. Milk production diminishes rapidly at this stage. There is usually a vaginal discharge, which smells offensively, and is discolored and watery (mostly thin and red-tinged).

(B) Pyometra. In addition to (A), the following symptoms are typical:
— Increased thirst
— A tense, distended belly, in which one can frequently feel the enlarged uterus
— Vaginal discharge, which is discolored depending on the causative agent. It is either greenish-yellow or muddy-red, and, in most cases, foul smelling.

Important: Immediate and specific treatment is essential to save the life of the animal.

Causes

(A) Premature births, and dead fetuses are the most frequent reasons for inflammatory problems of the uterus. Other causes are prolonged birthing complications, fetal anomalies, manual birthing assistance, and retained placentas.

(B) Pyometra may be the advanced stage of a primary inflammation. Another cause may be a disorder of the female hormone balance.

Hormone treatments and ovarian cysts create favorable conditions for the development of pyometra.

Self-Help
● Homeopathic Single Remedies
(A) If the condition develops slowly, and the cat does not show severe general disease, treat with the following two medications:

Use Pulsatilla 30C for 5 days if your cat is easy-going but shows varying moods, and if she is not thirsty, and the vaginal discharge is thick and creamy.

Use Sepia 30C, also for 5 days, if the queen shows a negative attitude toward her kittens, and if her vaginal secretion is of varying consistency.

(B) Pulsatilla 30C is the right treatment for a cuddly, moody cat, who has a suppurative vaginal discharge. Administer the medication twice daily, for 5 days, reducing to once daily for 5 days after recovery has begun.

For a cat who does not want to care for her kittens and whose secretion is discolored brown, Sepia 12X should be given for 10 days.

● Bach Flowers

Symptoms	Treatment
Sickness following delivery	Walnut
Lethargic and resigned	Wild Rose, Walnut
Weak and listless	Centaury
Internally unclean	Crab Apple
Tired, needing stimulus for strength	Hornbeam

● Combination Remedies
(A) For fever conditions following a birth, treat the queen with Febrisal for 4 days, mornings and evenings with ½ ampule each in the drinking water. Or you can dissolve it in water and place it directly into the mouth.

Or, you can treat her with Echinacea comp. S for 5 days, twice daily, with one ampule in the drinking water.

(B) The French school of classic homeopathy recommends the following: Mix equal parts of powders from Sepia 6X, Helonias 6X, and Hydrastis 6X (this should be done by the pharmacist), and administer one dose three times daily. Once improvement is noticeable, reduce the dosage until recovery is complete.

When to Get Professional Help
Both uterine diseases are serious illnesses and must be treated immediately by a veterinarian.

What Are the Treatment Options?
(A) A veterinarian trained in health care techniques will determine the suitability of a homeopathic treatment course. Otherwise, antibiotic and localized treatment of the uterus have to be initiated. It is also possible to administer a drug that contracts the uterus. If the cat is exhausted, e.g., following a difficult birth process, it will be necessary to give the animal strength through an intravenous infusion of electrolytes and glucose.

(B) As a rule, the treatment calls for an ovariohysterectomy, i.e., the removal of the ovaries, oviducts, and of the uterus.

Prevention and Convalescent Care
(A) Give your pregnant queen, in each of the last 2 weeks before she is due to deliver, one dose of Sepia 30C or Pulsatilla 30C according to her constitutional make-up.

If the animal turns out to have birthing complications it is a good idea to ask a veterinarian for a prophylactic treatment to prevent an ensuing uterine infection. Without this treatment the cat is likely to develop pyometra.

Cats who suffer from uterine inflammation usually do not have enough milk for the litter. Be prepared to feed the newborn kittens with additional mother replacement milk.

4

(B) You can prevent pyometra by having the cat spayed. If surgery is indicated the veterinarian will advise you of the correct postsurgical care. For directions on homeopathic postsurgical support see page 27.

Mastitis

An inflammation of the mammary glands is called mastitis. This condition happens because there are not enough kittens to drink all of the milk which causes it to remain in the tissues where it causes an inflammation. The same may happen if milk remains after the kittens have been weaned.

Symptoms
The mother cat is restless and tries to push away her kittens. The mammary glands appear red, hot, and swollen. The tissue feels hard, and is painful to touch. Often the cat develops a fever, appears lethargic, and does not eat or drink.

Causes
Bacteria find their way into the milk that is backed up inside the mammary glands. Here they multiply, which develops quickly into mastitis.

Self-Help
Cooling compresses are the most effective external method of reducing a painful mastitis. Here is a tried and proven procedure: Mix fruit vinegar with water 1:4, and use it for compresses three to four times daily.

Important: Pathogenic germs can be transmitted from the mother to the pups while they nurse. It is better to remove them from the sick queen and to feed them mother replacement milk.

● **Homeopathic Single Remedies**
Belladonna 12X is indicated for mastitis that appears suddenly, with high fever, and with acute reddening and swelling.

Apis 12X should be used when the mastitis looks more like a bee sting, the tissue is very sensitive to touch, it is edematous, and the cat does not drink anything at all.

Administer one dose of these medications every 2 hours during the acute phase, and alternate them if you are dealing with a particularly severe case.

Lachesis 12X is the right medication for a mastitis that is localized on one side, shows bluish discoloration, and which gets worse at night. Administer this three to six times daily during the acute stage, then reduce the dosage slowly.

● **Bach Flowers**

Symptoms	Treatment
Severe internal traumatization	Rescue Remedy
Apathy, resignation	Wild Rose
Inflammatory reaction	Holly

● **Combination Remedies**
Belladonna-Homaccord and Traumeel tablets will reduce the inflammation quickly, especially if you alternate their administration.

Dosages for all remedies are listed on the inside front cover.

Important: Treat the nursing queen until the mammary glands appear normal.

When to Get Professional Help

Get help from a veterinarian as soon as you suspect mastitis. This condition threatens the well-being of the mother and the lives of the kittens.

What Are the Treatment Options?

The first goal is to reduce the inflammatory process. Antibiotics and/or anti-inflammatory drugs may have to be administered by a veterinarian.

Prevention and Convalescent Care

If a cat does not have enough offspring for the amount of milk she is producing, she can be offered as a foster mother. Before you place orphans with the foster mother you would have to rub all kittens with a little alcohol in order to make them odor-neutral. Orphan kittens must be bottlefed every 2 to 3 hours, day and night, during the first week. Feeding is followed by a gentle massage of the belly and of the anal region to stimulate elimination (see raising orphan kittens on page 18).

4

Diseases of the Skin and Glands

The skin serves as a sensory organ with which to communicate with the world. It receives stimuli from the environment and transmits them to the brain. On the other hand the skin serves as a protective garment that prevents damaging influences like chemicals, radiation, heat, or mechanical impact from entering the body. The skin also regulates the body temperature and participates in the water and electrolyte balance. As soon as you notice changes in the appearance of the fur, or you notice itching, hair loss, or inflammation, you should examine the cat for parasites, scaly eruptions, or injuries. In addition skin problems may reflect an internal disease, like nephritis, hepatitis, or allergies.

The glands produce life-supporting hormones, which influence all metabolic pathways at the smallest concentration. The most significant glands are the hypophysis, the thyroid, pancreas, adrenals, and the gonads.

Glandular disease is rare in cats, and would require professional treatment if observed.

Abscesses

An abscess is an accumulation of pus inside an encapsulated hollow tissue. Prevalent locations are the head, chest, and tail.

Symptoms
An acutely inflamed area (abscess) is painful and warm to the touch. During the advanced stage of the condition the body temperature is increased, and the cat appears lethargic and exhausted. The climax of the infection is usually reached on the tenth to fourteenth day. Once the abscess breaks open the secretion will be colored according to the causative agent: watery-blood tinged, or thick and greenish. It is from this point on that the healing process begins.

Causes
Fights with territorial rivals lead to bites and scratches, which get infected with bacteria and dirt. After a few days the skin closes over the injury, and the bacteria continue to multiply under the skin, causing a productive inflammation. The body tries to control the trouble by encapsulating the inflammation, and by melting the bacterial agents with the dead cells; as a result, an abscess forms.

Self-Help
Topical treatment with an acetate mixture is indicated. Use it to prepare a poultice, which you place twice daily on the abscessed area to achieve cooling of the inflammation, and to reduce the pain.

● **Homeopathic Single Remedies**
In the beginning stages, Hepar sulfuris 12X will heal an abscess in the early stages, by stimulating the body to resolve the abscess internally.

If you are dealing with an encapsulated abscess, which you want to induce to open up, treat the cat with Hepar sulfuris 6X for 7 days.

Once the abscess is open, the administration of Silica 12X, given over 8 days, will complete the healing process.

● Bach Flowers
If the defenses of your cat are weakened give the animal Centaury, and choose Crab Apple to induce an internal cleansing. You may use both flower preparations at the same time.

● Combination Remedies
Administer one tablet Traumeel, alternating with Mercurius-Heel, three to six times daily. Apply a pain relieving coat of Traumeel or Rescue Remedy ointment externally.

Dosages for all remedies are listed on the inside front cover.

When to Get Professional Help
Get professional help if your treatments are unsuccessful, or if the cat's general well-being is affected.

What Are the Treatment Options?
If necessary, the veterinarian could puncture the abscess to determine a causative agent. A well-developed abscess is opened surgically.

Prevention and Convalescent Care
Fighting between rival cats is hard to avoid. If you have a repeat offender, who comes home with cuts and bruises, you should get the cat spayed/neutered (page 19).

Phlegmon

Phlegmons (page 121) are infections of the connective tissue, which occur mainly along the limbs.

Symptoms
Pathogens have entered through the opening of a small wound. The spot is now swollen, red, warm, and painful. If the inflammation is allowed to spread, there will be general symptoms of illness. The cat might limp on the affected side. If the condition progresses, pain will prevent the animal from using the limb altogether. Even a touch of the paw elicits severe pain.

Causes
Skin lesions that are caused by accidents or by bites allow pathogens to enter the subcutaneous tissues. Here, the germs multiply. In most cases, these are bacterial pathogens, which cause the formation of pus.

Self-Help
For the cooling of the warm swelling you should prepare twice daily a poultice soaked in a mixture of water and vinegar (3:1).

● Homeopathic Single Remedies
During the first 3 to 5 days administer daily three alternating doses of Belladonna 6X and Apis 6X, one dose every 2 hours. As soon as improvement sets in reduce the doses to one each per day, until the phlegmon is healed.

If an abscess forms follow directions on page 68.

● **Bach Flowers**

Symptoms	Treatment
Lesion after injury	Rescue Remedy
Diminished resistance	Centaury
Unclean condition	Crab Apple
Painful inflammation	Holly

● **Combination Remedies**

To reduce the severe and painful inflammation of a phlegmon administer Belladonna-Homaccord three to six times daily, or Belladonna, alternating with Traumeel, three doses daily.

Another treatment which helps in cases of these inflammatory lesions is Echinacea comp. S. Administer daily ½ ampule in the drinking water, or give it via a disposable syringe directly into the mouth.

Dosages for all remedies are listed on the inside front cover.

When to Get Professional Help

Phlegmons are often discovered only after signs of limping or general symptoms appear. Unless your home treatments show quick results, you should consult a veterinarian.

What Are the Treatment Options?

The type of natural remedies that will be chosen to treat a phlegmon depend on the following: the general condition of the cat; the degree of inflammatory swelling; and the degree to which the joints are in danger of being infected. If the condition cannot be calmed completely, it may be necessary to add an antibiotic treatment to the regimen.

Prevention and Convalescent Care

In every case of injury you should first administer Arnica 12X. This will set the scene for healing.

If an allopathic course of treatment is indicated (page 120), the administration of Sulfur 30C will rebalance the organism after the healing is complete.

Acne

A cat's chin has an accumulation of follicles that have a tendency to become inflamed (folliculitis).

Symptoms

The chin appears swollen, and the skin is red and painful. The hair falls out because the secretion of the follicles cakes up. In most cases there are small pustules or pimples, or red areas enlarge and develop pus, which indicates that an extensive inflammation of the hair follicles has occurred.

Causes

Bacteria enter the hair follicles, where they cause a suppurative inflammatory reaction. Internal problems, such as a hormonal imbalance, can also lead to acne.

Self-Help

Clean the external surface gently with chamomile tea, and follow three times daily with a thin coat of Calendula or Traumeel ointment.

● **Homeopathic Single Remedies**

Administer Hepar sulfuris 12X for 1 to 2 weeks.

● **Bach Flowers**

To treat the topical inflammation use Crab Apple; to increase internal defenses administer Walnut.

● **Combination Remedies**
Treat your cat with Traumeel tablets.

Dosages for all remedies are listed on the inside front cover.

When to Get Professional Help
If the acne is accompanied by other signs of illness, it would be advisable to get a blood analysis done. This would determine the existence of any potential organic disorders.

Prevention and Convalescent Care
If your cat appears to be predisposed for acne it is a good idea to check the chin area regularly, and to treat the condition in its early stages.

Hair Loss

Cats shed their coat "normally" twice yearly, which is a seasonal adaptation to spring and fall. Hair loss in circumscribed areas, and increased shedding outside of the normal seasons, suggests an illness.

Symptoms
The pattern of hair loss may range from small round spots to large areas. The appearance is usually typical for the cause.

Gastritis and vomiting of hair balls (page 51) may follow as a consequence of the increased ingestion of hair during grooming.

Causes
There are a number of external causes for hair loss (alopecia): Ectoparasites (pages 84–86), fungal infections (page 96), dermatitis and eczema (page 72), as well as contact and flea allergies.

Internal causes for alopecia are organ diseases (e.g., liver, kidney), food allergies, bacterial infections (e.g., tuberculosis), tapeworm infestation, or hormonal imbalances. In addition, heredity plays a part in hair loss, as well as exposure to stress or to infectious diseases.

Important: Pay special attention to local areas of hair loss in varying patterns, because you need to consider causes that are potentially transmissible to humans.

Self-Help
● **Homeopathic Single Remedies**
If the hair loss occurs following a spay/neuter treat the cat with Staphisagria 12X for 7 days.

If, however, the fur appears dull, soiled, and smelly, Sulfur 30C, given for 7 days, will be most effective.

● **Bach Flowers**

Symptoms	Treatment
Soiled, dull fur	Crab Apple
Worsening condition	Wild Rose
Exhaustion	Olive
Allergic reaction	Beech

● **Combination Remedies**
Sulfur-Heel is best for skin allergies and chronic skin problems. You might want to give it alternatingly with Traumeel, giving daily two tablets each. If the hair loss occurs in combination with other skin diseases you should choose Cutis comp. of which you administer one ampule, one to three times per week, in the drinking water.

Dosages for all remedies are listed on the inside front cover.

5

When to Get Professional Help

All hair loss is caused by an underlying disorder. This should be determined by a professional caregiver, even if your home treatment appears to be effective.

What Are the Treatment Options?

Typical diagnostic methods would include a skin scraping, a blood test, and a stool analysis.

For the enhancement of the overall condition of the cat the veterinarian will select a specific constitutional remedy (page 119).

Prevention and Convalescent Care

Regular worm treatments (page 16) and optimal nutrition (page 12) are the best insurance for a healthy fur coat. You can prevent the excessive ingestion of hair by thorough brushing sessions during the shedding cycles.

Check your cat regularly for parasites (page 84), especially during warm seasons.

Important: A cat's fur is like a barometer for the overall condition of the animal. The disease which underlies the appearance of hair loss must therefore be treated with great care.

Eczema

Eczema is an inflammatory condition of the skin, which can appear in many forms. It is often aggravated by the cat's habit of licking, which introduces bacterial infections into the area. Feline eczema presents an often stubborn problem in the practice setting. These conditions are often quite resistant to treatment, and must be evaluated carefully for any potential underlying causes.

Symptoms

The first signals for eczema are usually hair loss (page 71), increased licking in a particular area, and a general sense of restlessness. More or less severe itching is a typical problem, which often causes the cat to bite and scratch continuously. This, in turn, causes the animal increasing pain, until it becomes nearly impossible to touch. As an affected area enlarges the symptoms worsen.

Depending on the appearance of the form of eczema, one refers to papules, pustules, vesicles, or patches of crusts. If the inflammation has spread, the eczema may appear dry, or seeping-moist, or crusty and scaly.

The appearance of the skin change is indicative for the choice of natural remedies.

Causes

The external causes for eczema are parasites (pages 84–89), contact and chemical allergies (e.g., flea collars), as well as mechanical injuries, and chemical or physical irritations. Viruses, bacteria, and fungi may cause eczema as secondary infectious agents.

Internal causes for eczema are inadequate diets, endoparasites (pages 87–89), as well as metabolic and intestinal disorders (page 51). Food allergies and diabetes may also cause this condition.

Self-Help

Important: Before you begin home treatment be sure to check the last date of worm treatment.

If you have been feeding a monotonous diet, change the food now (page 12). Cats who are fed predominantly with dry food are more likely to suffer from skin disorders.

Topical treatments with Calendula ointment or drops, or with Saint John's Wort oil take away the itch and have a calming effect on the skin irritation.

● Homeopathic Single Remedies

Sulfur 12X is the right choice if the skin appears dry and scaly, with itching eczema, which is aggravated by scratching and grooming. The cat smells bad, and so do its excreta. The body orifices are red and inflamed, and the cat seeks cold places because its body temperature is high.

Natrium muriaticum 12X is for cats who are shy and scared and who are easily tired. This eczema is mainly found in the areas of joints, where it forms red and itching spots. An eczema that secretes a thick, honey-like substance must be treated with Graphites 12X. These cats are usually overweight, sleepy, and hungry all day long.

Mercurius is most effective for moist eczema with blisters, or with pus-filled pustules. The skin appears ulcerated, the scabs form pus, and salivation is often increased, especially at night.

If the eczema is dry, scaly, and chronic, Arsenicum 12X will heal the skin. Itching and burning are typical Arsenicum symptoms. Noteworthy is the pattern of nightly aggravation of this form of eczema. Also, these animals seek warmth, and they are very thirsty, but drink only tiny amounts.

The worst cases of itching, combined with bad body and secretory odors, are treated with the nosode Psorinum 12X. These cats are usually sensitive to cold temperatures. Psorinum should be chosen, also, if none of the other remedies are fully successful.

All of the above remedies should be administered twice daily until the eczema is healed.

● Bach Flowers

Symptoms	Treatment
Unthrifty, dull coat	Crab Apple
Hypersensitive skin reactions	Beech
Lowered defense abilities	Centaury
"Exhausted" skin condition	Olive

● Combination Remedies

Schwef-Heel drops or Sulfur-Heel tablets are most helpful for itching eczema and similar skin eruptions. If, however, your cat is well-nourished, is always ready to eat, and suffers from dry, scaly, broken skin conditions, you should treat your pet with Graphites-Homaccord.

Dosages for all remedies are located on the inside front cover.

When to Get Professional Help

If your cat's skin does not improve with treatment, and if it appears to be suffering from its condition you should consult a veterianarian.

What Are the Treatment Options?

A skin scraping will be the most effective method to exclude any external causes. If an internal problem is suspected it is necessary to check blood, urine, and stool.

If the fur appears sticky, caked, or with crusty scabs, the veterinarian will clip the hair away from the most affected areas, so that the underlying skin can dry and heal with the appropriate treatments. Ointments and powders may be considered; however, they are often too dense in their coverage. In many cases it may be better to treat the "whole animal" because the skin condition has become an expression of internal organic imbalance.

Prevention and Convalescent Care

Inappropriate diet is frequently a cause of eczema. Offer your cat a well-balanced, varied meal plan (page 12). If your cat appears to have particular skin sensitivities it is best to eliminate dry foods. Never feed your cat dog food. You may want to buy special diets that are formulated for skin sensitivities.

Regular tapeworm treatments are especially important for outdoor cats and for those cats who come in contact with other cats or with feral rodents. For ectoparasites see pages 84–88.

Make sure that all household chemicals are out of reach of a curious kitten. Internal disorders must be thoroughly treated until they are completely cured. It is only in this way that you can prevent secondary involvement of other organs, like the skin.

Important: Eczema conditions must be treated according to the directions of the veterinarian until the cat has grown a healthy shiny new fur coat. Be prepared for this to take weeks or months.

Tumors

Tumors are seen more often in old cats than in young ones. Tumors may occur singly or in varying numbers.

Benign tumors are typically well circumscribed, can be moved over the underlying tissue, occur singly, and usually do not change shape and consistency over prolonged time periods.

Malignant tumors, as a rule, grow quickly, and invade the underlying tissues, making them hard to move and to define in their location. They are spread via the lymph or blood vessels to other organ systems. In cases of malignant tumors the cat's general condition often worsens as the tumor grows.

Symptoms
(A) Tumors of the skin appear as knot-like enlargements. It is common for cats not to show any symptoms of illness for a prolonged time.

(B) Mammary gland tumors appear prevalently as a row of irregular enlargements along the line of the nipples. They are usually painless, and take a long time to grow. However, they can quite suddenly start growing very rapidly, thus causing the cat more and more discomfort.

Causes
The cause of cancer is scientifically not explained. Some viral participation has been postulated. Environment, climate, and heredity may contribute to cancer development, as well as nutrition and infectious diseases.

Self-Help
Tumors of the skin and mammary glands can be externally supported by treatments with Traumeel or with Calendula ointment.

● **Homeopathic Single Remedies**
(A) and (B) Use Conium 12X for hard, painful, and knotty tumors. Administer it three times daily during the first week, continue with twice daily doses.

(A) Thuja 12X is the right medication for warts or wart-like skin growths.

Calcium carbonicum 30C and Lycopodium 30C are also helpful for tumors of the skin. Give five globules of either substance once daily for 1 week, if the substance fits the cat's constitutional pattern (page 120).

(B) Phytolacca 6X is the right medication for mammary tumors that are hard and painful. The tumor may lead to inflammation and abscesses. Administer Phytolacca during the acute phase six times daily, then three times daily for several weeks.

● **Bach Flowers**

Symptoms	Treatment
Condition unchanged	Wild Oat
Tiredness, especially mornings	Hornbeam
Lowered vitality	Scleranthus
Restlessness	Agrimony
Suffering from tumors	Holly

If your cat appears tired, apathetic, and behaves with indifference, then give it a mixture of Wild Oat, Hornbeam, and Scleranthus.

● **Combination Remedies**

Carcinomium comp. helps with tumors of the skin and mammary glands. Give $1/2$ ampule every third day in the drinking water. This treatment should be planned and supervised by a veterinarian.

Dosages for all remedies are listed on the inside front cover.

When to Get Professional Help

Tumors in general, and fast growing ones particularly, should be examined by a veterinarian.

What Are the Treatment Options?

Natural holistic treatment methods have proved to be effective in reducing or eliminating mammary gland tumors.

As long as a tumor is small, and hardly visible, it is only necessary to watch its development. When the location or size of the tumor visibly causes discomfort, it must be removed surgically. For directions on postsurgical care see page 27.

Prevention and Convalescent Care

(A) Skin tumors occur only rarely in cats, and they are predominantly benign. Observe any small knots in the skin, and show them to your veterinarian at the next vaccination appointment.

(B) While you brush and pet your cat examine the mammary glands from time to time, checking for any abnormalities. Small knots are not necessarily cancerous. Glandular tissue may harden, or form cysts—neither being serious problems. Your health care practitioner will advise you how best to manage the condition.

Hyperthyroidism

The thyroid gland is located on either side of the larynx at the sides of the neck. You cannot feel this gland, unless it is abnormally enlarged and overproducing.

Symptoms

The characteristic sign for a thyroid gland that is overproducing thyroid hormone is an increased activity of many body functions. Emaciation occurs, despite increased hunger, because the food is not properly digested in the overactive intestinal tract. Large-formed, frequent stools are symptomatic. Sometimes diarrhea occurs. Cats may become frightened easily, their heart rate increases, and the pulse becomes irregular. Obvious thirst is typical, as is an occasional muscular weakness and trembling.

Causes

The majority of hyperthyroidism are caused by benign enlargements of the gland. Cancer is very rare.

5

Self-Help
● Homeopathic Single Remedies
Jodum 30C (Iodine 30C) should be given over 2 weeks. This substance is specific for this condition, as iodine is a component of the thyroid hormone. Once the condition has improved you may repeat the treatment after a 1 week interval.

● Bach Flowers

Symptoms	Treatment
Restlessness, nervous weight loss	Impatiens
Exhaustion	Olive

● Combination Remedies
You will improve the condition of your cat by giving it three times daily five to ten drops of Lymphomyosot.

Dosages for all remedies are listed on the inside front cover.

When to Get Professional Help
A veterinarian must be consulted throughout this treatment.

What Are the Treatment Options?
Palpation would reveal an enlargement of the thyroid gland. A blood test is analyzed to determine the amount of thyroid hormone being produced.

If natural remedies are not effective in reducing the hormone production it is necessary to use allopathic treatments to lower it.

Surgical removal of the gland is another promising treatment alternative.

Prevention and Convalescent Care
This sick cat needs much tender care and support. Optimal care combined with excellent choices of natural remedies greatly improve the prognostic outlook.

Pancreatitis

The pancreas produces digestive enzymes, which help process proteins, fats, and carbohydrates. The pancreatic "islets" are the cell complexes in which insulin is produced. Insulin regulates the blood sugar levels. Pancreatitis, an inflammation of the pancreas, is a rare condition in the cat. The acute form is usually unrecognized because it does not cause specific symptoms. When it occurs, pancreatitis is mostly found in the chronic form.

Symptoms
An acute pancreatitis is mainly expressed by general signs, like vomiting and diarrhea, and a tense belly because of pain. If left untreated the condition develops into a chronic pancreatitis.

While the cat may show increased appetite in the beginning stages of the disease, it will soon develop into loss of appetite, general weakness, and weight loss. The digestive process is disturbed, expressing itself in diarrhea, sometimes constipation, flatulence, and vomiting. Noteworthy is the typically glistening, fatty, light gray stool, which is eliminated more frequently than normal and in higher volumes. Unusual is also the high frequency and volume of drinking, and of urination.

Causes
The cause of pancreatitis is not clear. It is possible that pathogens from the digestive tract can reach the pancreas and cause the inflammation.

Self-Help

Important: The treatment must be initiated by a professional health care practitioner. The suggested remedies may be used in conjunction with the main medications.

● **Homeopathic Single Remedies**

If the cat loses weight despite a voracious appetite, administer Jodum 30C.

Give the animal five globules twice daily, for 5 days, then reduce to once daily for the next 10 days. Jodum 12X may also be used.

An alternative course of treatment, developed by Wolff, specifies medicating the cat for an extended period with Haronga 4X and Iris versicolor 6X, three globules each, before meals.

Chionanthus 12X is indicated for cats who eliminate stool that is clay-colored to yellow-creamy-soft, and who urinate frequently. The urine is usually darkly colored and contains sugar. Medicate this cat twice daily, five globules each time, for 2 to 3 weeks.

The nosode Pancreatinum 30C, given once daily, for 1 week, may be administered in combination with other treatments.

● **Bach Flowers**

Symptoms	Treatment
Restless behavior	Agrimony
Increasing weakness	Gentian
Severe tiredness and exhaustion	Olive

● **Combination Remedies**

The main medication for chronic pancreatitis is Leptandra comp. Depending on the other symptoms Leptandra should be combined with the following medications:

– Bryaconeel, if peritonitis and liver enlargement are diagnosed.

– Chelidonium Homaccord, for liver and gallbladder disorders.

– Spascupreel, when abdominal pain is apparent.

– Duodenoheel, where emaciation coexists with unabridged hunger, and with colitis.

– Cardiacum-Heel for cases of circulatory problems.

Dosages for all remedies are listed on the inside front cover.

When to Get Professional Help

Consult a veterinarian if you notice large formed, light-colored stools. These are serious signs of disease.

What Are the Treatment Options?

If you are dealing with a cat in the acute stage of the disease you can reduce the inflammatory process by fasting the cat, and placing it subsequently on a specific diet. During this stage the cat should be receiving intravenous nutrients from a veterinarian.

In order to assess the degree of severity of the condition and to determine the prognosis for organ regeneration it is necessary to analyze the stool, blood, and urine. This will lead to a specific diet and remedy selection.

If it turns out that the cat suffers from diabetes, it will be necessary to add insulin to the course of medications.

Prevention and Convalescent Care

As your cat gets older you should check the stool consistency more frequently, and you should have a good idea about the amount of drinking water that is being consumed.

Cats who suffer from a chronic pancreatitis should be fed a special diet, which is formulated to support a disturbed digestive system. If you prepare the food at home you can supplement it by adding powdered enzymes, which predigest the nutrient components.

5

Diseases of the Musculoskeletal and Nervous Systems

Mobility is a cat's essential characteristic. Muscles, tendons, bones, and joints work in total harmony when a cat trains its body in play, running, chasing, climbing, or hunting prey. The brain receives these stimuli via the nerves, processes them, and transforms them into appropriate reactions.

When any of the involved organs are damaged or destroyed the cat must deal with significant restrictions.

Injuries of the Musculoskeletal System

When joints, tendons, or muscles are pulled or turned beyond their physiological tension point a distortion, or sprain occurs. In the worst case a tear would occur. A luxation refers to a condition where the joint capsule, muscles, and tendons, as well as vessels are torn apart. A contusion occurs if muscles or tissues are hit by blunt force. This lesion is usually marked by a painful swelling.

Symptoms
The cat will limp more or less severely depending on the degree of injury and pain. The affected leg is used barely, or not at all. The joint or other affected area is most commonly swollen and warm to the touch.

Causes
Most cases are caused by jumps or falls from windows, by car accidents, or by forceful kicks or blows with a stick.

Self-Help
For an acute injury, take the animal to a quiet location, cover it with a blanket, and examine it gently for cuts and bleeding. For directions see pages 108 and 112.

● **Homeopathic Single Remedies**
Arnica 12X is indicated for all kinds of injuries. Begin with five globules every 30 minutes, administered in water, directly into the mouth. From the second day on alternate the Arnica treatment with Rhus toxicodendron 12X. Give five globules every 2 hours for 4 days. After this you continue with Rhus toxicodedron alone, two to three times each day until the cat is well.

● **Bach Flowers**
Rescue Remedy is indicated for all kinds of accidents, injuries, and shock.

Dosages for all remedies are listed on the inside front cover.

● **Combination Remedies**
Give one Traumeel tablet three to six times daily during the first few days, and reduce the treatment as the cat improves.

When to Get Professional Help

If your cat could be seriously hurt it is best to ask for a professional checkup.

What Are the Treatment Options?

An injection of a strong analgesic will reduce the pain quickly and speed recovery. In addition, a bandage can often reduce the burden on an injured limb.

Prevention and Convalescent Care

Accidents can happen. Therefore it is best to be prepared by stocking the right treatments: Arnica 12X and Rescue Remedy.

Arthritis

Acute or chronic inflammatory conditions of a joint are referred to as arthritis; chronic degenerative joint disease is called arthrosis. Arthrosis in the cat is very rare, and would have to be diagnosed by x-ray.

Symptoms

As a rule the acute form of arthritis affects only one joint. Its signs are warmth, swelling, and pain. The cat will favor the limb, and avoid movement.

The chronic form of arthritis is characterized by limping, while pain and swelling are mostly absent.

Causes

Joint inflammation may be caused by injuries, with or without tearing of the capsule. Generalized infectious diseases can also cause joint disease.

Self-Help

If an injury is the cause of the problem, give Arnica 12X and proceed as indicated on page 78.

In order to promote healing and to reduce the painful swelling place a compress soaked in water with vinegar (mixed 4:1), on the affected limb. Or, you can use an Acetate mixture (mixed by the pharmacist) in the same way.

● Homeopathic Single Remedies

For the treatment of a hot joint you need to administer Bryonia 12X, alternating with Rhus toxicodendron 12X every 2 hours. As soon as you observe improvement, reduce the dosage to twice daily until recovery is complete.

For chronic cases of arthritis choose Bryonia 12X for 10 to 14 days if your cat gets worse with increased movement. If, however, mobility improves the condition, then Rhus toxicodendron 12X is indicated.

● Bach Flowers

Symptoms	Treatment
Symptoms caused by accident	Rescue Remedy
Severe inflammation	Holly
Restless, nervous	Agrimony

● Combination Remedies

In all cases of injuries you should administer one tablet of Traumeel three to six times daily.

In cases of arthrosis the practitioner is likely to begin the treatment with an injection of Zeel, which you will continue at home by giving Zeel tablets orally.

Dosages for all remedies are listed on the inside front cover.

6

When to Get Professional Help

Professional advice is urgently needed if your home treatments have not shown visible improvement within 2 days.

What Are the Treatment Options?

If home remedies have not improved the condition it would be best to have the animal treated with anti-inflammatory drugs.

Prevention and Convalescent Care

Injuries are hard to prevent. Be prepared by keeping your medicine chest stocked with Arnica, Rescue Remedy, or Saint John's Wort.

If your cat suffers from acutely affected joints, keep the animal quiet.

Bone Fractures

Bones break when their tension capacity is exceeded. The most frequent fractures are located in the jaws, limbs, pelvis, and ribs. A cat's bones heal exceptionally well, rarely requiring surgery. In cases of closed fractures the skin remains closed, while open fractures are visible through the broken skin.

Symptoms

Important: Fractures are extremely painful. These cats require a most gentle touch, and should be moved with the greatest care.

Fractures are usually characterized by abnormally positioned limbs, by protruding bones, by excessive swelling following an accident, and by the sound of crepitation, i.e., the sound of bone fragments rubbing together during an examination.

Causes

Fractures are mostly caused by accidents with cars or by falling from balconies or windows.

Self-Help

Home remedies are administered in addition to the veterinary treatment regimen.

● **Homeopathic Single Remedies**

Arnica 12X should be given following any injury.

For the stimulation of callus formation, Symphytum 2X is indicated at five globules, four times, as well as Calcium phosphoricum 8X, five globules mornings and evenings. Both medications should be continued until the bones are fully healed.

● **Bach Flowers**

Bone fractures call for the administration of Rescue Remedy.

● **Combination Remedies**

During the first few days give your cat one Traumeel tablet three to six times daily, then reduce to three times daily.

Dosages for all remedies are listed on the inside front cover.

When to Get Professional Help

An injured cat with a fracture needs to be seen by a veterinarian.

What Are the Treatment Options?

Veterinary care will first provide for a stabilized circulatory system, and alleviate any shock symptoms. Subsequently the animal will have x-rays in order to establish the treatment plan. The corrective treatment options for fractures are either conservative or surgical.

Conservative correction implies the alignment of the bones and their stabilization with external alignments and bandages or with casts. Cats do not tolerate casts well.

Surgical correction is mostly chosen for complex fractures. Fractures of the upper front and hindlegs are also better corrected with surgical techniques because these bones are weight bearing. In this procedure the bones are fixed in alignment by screws, nails, plates, or wires, which are removed after the healing is complete.

Regular bandage changes are part of the post-surgical care program at the veterinary hospital. Certain injections to promote bone growth and to reduce swelling might also be indicated. If it is likely that the fracture was contaminated the cat would receive antibiotics.

Important: Amputation is necessary if the injured bones were completely crushed in the accident, or if the injury is old. Cats compensate well for the loss of a limb, and will soon be able to climb objects.

Prevention and Convalescent Care

Follow the instructions of the veterinarian.

If a cat appears too restless, you may need to restrain the animal either by fitting it with an Elizabethan collar or by restricting its movement in a cage (page 113).

Paralysis

When a nerve is damaged the area around it turns numb and loses sensitivity. Cats suffer specifically from nerve injuries of the front paw, and from injuries caused by a window closing across their back, leaving them hemiplegic.

Symptoms

If the front paw is paralyzed the cat pulls the paw along the floor. The paw appears loose and lifeless.

If the cat was injured by a window falling on its back, it is no longer able to walk and will have to drag its hindquarters along the floor. Due to the nerve damage there is no pain associated with this condition.

Causes

Most cases of paralysis are caused by accidents.

Self-Help

Tender loving care is the essential ingredient in caring for a paralyzed cat.

● **Homeopathic Single Remedies**

On the first day of injury give your cat Arnica 12X, five globules every 2 hours. Give it directly into the mouth or put 20 globules in the daily drinking water. You may also choose a higher potency, e.g., 30C, four times on the first day.

On the second day you begin to alternate the Arnica treatment with Hypericum 12X. Now, for 1 week, the paralyzed patient receives Arnica three times daily and Hypericum 12X three times daily (i.e., every 2 hours). After 1 week you continue with Hypericum alone, twice daily, until the animal is well.

● **Bach Flowers**

Rescue Remedy and Star of Bethlehem are the right flowers for injuries.

Dosages are listed on the inside front cover.

6

● **Combination Remedies**

During the first week give the animal one Traumeel tablet three to six times daily, then reduce to three tablets per day.

When to Get Professional Help

Following a serious accident take your cat to veterinary clinic immediately. Directions for transporting the cat are on page 108. Get professional help if your home remedies are not showing significant improvement.

What Are the Treatment Options?

The veterinarian will first stabilize the heart, and then treat shock symptoms and replace body fluids by an intravenous infusion. B vitamins will be added to rebuild nerve tissue.

It may be necessary to take x-rays of the vertebral column and limbs in order to assess recovery expectations.

Prevention and Convalescent Care

The prospect of recovering damaged nerve cells and nerves is not hopeless. Patience, persistence, as well as quiet rest, warmth, and tender loving care are the main ingredients of treatment. Watching your cat recover will be your greatest reward.

Disorders of the Mineral Metabolism

Cats suffer only occasionally from mineral disorders. When bone building is disturbed, it leads to rickets in kittens, and to osteomalacia in older cats.

Symptoms

The cat appears to limp without any obvious reason. Kittens may be diagnosed with excessive bone growth on the end of the long bones, e.g., the upper hindlegs, while their overall growth is behind normal expectations. It may also develop as rosary-like bony growths along the ribs, or in crippling deformations of the limbs.

Causes

Mineral disorders may be caused by poor nutrition, lack of minerals or vitamin D, by lack of exposure to sunlight, or by hormonal disorders.

Some cats have a hereditary disposition to rickets. For these cats constitutional remedies are highly effective.

Self-Help

● **Homeopathic Single Remedies**

Kittens with growth disorders should be treated with Calcium phosphoricum 12X for 2 to 3 weeks.

Older cats who are heavier should receive 14 days of Calcium carbonicum 12X, or 7 days of Calcium carbonicum 30X to achieve deep healing. If this does not yield improvement, pause for 2 weeks, then administer Calcium phosphoricum 12X for 3 weeks.

● **Bach Flowers**

Chestnut Bud will aid a kitten that develops too slowly.

● **Combination Remedies**

Alternate between Calcoheel and Osteoheel, giving one tablet each, twice daily for 2 to 3 weeks.

Dosages for all remedies are listed on the inside front cover.

When to Get Professional Help

Get a veterinarian's help if your cat does *not* show any improvement after your treatment.

What Are the Treatment Options?

A blood test will help the veterinarian establish the correct treatment. Part of the necessary medications will be calcium/phosphorus as well as vitamin D.

Prevention and Convalescent Care

A monotonous meat diet may lead to mineral disorders in kittens. Changing the diet will be essential, e.g., reducing the meat component, while increasing the amount of vegetables, milk, and dry food. Commercially available foods are the best choice because they contain all necessary nutrients in the right proportions. Predisposed cats should be supplemented with minerals and vitamin D.

Important: Kittens who suffer from rickets may not be suitable for later breeding because they will pass the disposition on to their offspring.

Breed Disposition

Siamese cats show rickets more frequently than other breeds.

6

Parasitic Diseases

Parasites live and reproduce either inside or on the surface of their host. They damage their host by removing blood and other nutrients, while depositing their excrement, and causing inflammation.

Parasites that live in or on the skin are called ectoparasites (e.g., fleas, mites, and ticks), while endoparasites live inside the body of the host. Within the group of endoparasites there is a special enteric group (roundworms, hookworms, and tapeworms), which live in the gastrointestinal tract. These parasites damage the cat by withdrawing essential nutrients, thus rendering the animal more susceptible to other diseases, like respiratory infections or leukemia.

Fleas

Fleas live in the fur of the cat. Female fleas begin laying eggs soon after their first blood meal. Under favorable conditions flea eggs mature to adult stages within 3 weeks. Under unfavorable conditions it might take as long as 1 year.

The flea population is usually highest during late summer and early fall.

Symptoms
The cat scratches incessantly. You can see small dark crumbs of flea excrement, and sometimes fleas are obvious. Frequently there are rows of badly itching flea bites that can extend into large inflamed areas. Because of the continued scratching the hair will fall out. Repeated flea infestation may lead to hypersensitivity, which in turn causes an allergic flea eczema.

If kittens are severely infested with fleas they will lose weight, suffer from dermatitis, and develop anemia.

Important: Fleas are the intermediary hosts for tapeworm. Therefore it is necessary to consider a worm treatment after your cat has had fleas.

Causes
Cats contract cat fleas (*Ctenocephalides felis*) mainly from other cats, but fleas from dogs and hedgehogs will also bite cats.

Self-Help
Fleas detest your cat's fur if you brush and comb it regularly, and if you introduce scented oils into the fur.

● **Homeopathic Single Remedies**
As a rule fleas will attack the same animals over and over again. In such cases it is best to tune the body into a different mode with the help of a homeopathic single remedy. The following remedy will induce the fleas to avoid the cat: Administer Sulfur 30C, five globules every fifth day, for 4 weeks. Do this especially during the flea season. You can repeat this treatment after about 10 to 14 days.

● **Bach Flowers**
Crab Apple is the flower for cleansing. You can use Crab Apple in addition to the re-tuning of the body by adding 10 drops of the mother tincture in 8 oz. (½ L) bath water.

When to Get Professional Help

If your cat is heavily infested with fleas you should get veterinary help.

What Are the Treatment Options?

Veterinary consultation will help you choose the most suitable treatment. A number of options are available: Powders, shampoos, collars, liquids, baths, and tablets. In addition "Program" and "Advantage" are also available. Both are highly effective treatments that are given orally or topically once a month. They are as effective in combating fleas as they are easy to administer.

Important: Persian cats are hypersensitive to dichlorvos, and, therefore, should not be fitted with a flea collar.

Prevention and Convalescent Care

Sulfur 30C is indicated in cases of heavy flea infestation (see Self-Help section). While flea collars are a very effective prevention, they are known to cause allergic reactions. If your cat is allergic, you need to choose another method of flea control. Thoroughly clean all of the bedding and the resting areas where your cat likes to sleep with an insect repellent. This must be repeated because of the various maturation stages of the fleas. Check the animal and its bedding carefully for several weeks until you are sure that your plan was successful.

Mites

Mites are microscopically small parasites. Like spiders, they have four pairs of legs. Mites cause a group of disorders that are referred to as mange.

Mites of the Sarcoptes family take 10 to 14 days to undergo their maturation from egg through larval and nymph stages, to the adult mite. Ear mites and *Notoedres cati* take 21 days to mature. Mites live on or in the skin, and feed on body fluids and dead cell products.

Symptoms and Causes

(A) Ear mange (*parasitic otitis externa*) is caused by the ear mite *Otodectes cynotis:* The mites cause severe irritation and inflammation of the ear (page 37).

(B) Mange caused by Sarcoptes and *Notoedres cati:* The head area begins to show scaly crusts that extend first to the ears, and eventually over the whole body. The itching lesions keep the animal scratching relentlessly, and secondary infections set in. Allergic reactions may also complicate the condition.

(C) Grass mites (*Neotrombicula autumnalis*): After an outing on a beautiful autumn day your cat starts to scratch ferociously, particularly in the body areas with the least hair, such as the ears, between the toes, belly, inner thighs, chest, and genitalia. On closer examination you can see tiny bright red spots. These are the larvae of the grass mites. Because these mites usually invade in very large numbers, the cat suffers immensely from the excessive itching and inflammation (dermatitis).

Self-Help

(A) For self-help see page 37.

For (B) and (C) dab the affected areas with 10% Calendula solution.

● **Homeopathic Single Remedies**

Sulfur 12x is effective for treating lesions from mange mites as well as from grass mites. Administer it for 2 to 3 weeks, and repeat it if necessary after a pause between treatments.

7

● **Bach Flowers**

In cases (B) and (C) Crab Apple will be useful for an internal and external cleansing treatment (see "fleas", on page 84).

● **Combination Remedies**

Schwef-Heel, five drops, twice daily, should be given directly via a disposable syringe or via the drinking water.

Dosages for all remedies are listed on the inside front cover.

When to Get Professional Help

Consult a veterinarian if your home remedies have not yielded recovery after 1 to 2 weeks.

What Are the Treatment Options?

For ear mange (A) see page 37.

For (B) and (C) the veterinarian will take a skin scraping to analyze the type of mite that is involved.

If the animal is only mildly infested the treatment could be a topical treatment with any of several mite-killing chemicals. Since so many cats are notoriously fearful of baths, a spray or powder product may be easier to apply.

If you are dealing with a severely affected animal, where the whole body is itching and covered with lesions, the only reliable treatment is an injection with a specific drug against this condition. It must be administered by a veterinarian.

Prevention and Convalescent Care

If your cat roams around regularly you will need to give it equally regular parasite examinations.

If the animal is highly susceptible you should increase its resistance with treatments of Sulfur 30X, or with Bach Flowers, like Crab Apple, in order to modify the body's fine tuning.

Any treatment should be accompanied by a thorough cleaning of the cat's belongings, including blankets, pillows, etc.

Important: Once you have reason to suspect mange in your cat you need to act knowledgeably, specifically, and immediately. Isolate the affected cat from any other cats because it is very infectious. Since mange may also affect humans it is important to perform all cleaning tasks in the most hygienic method.

Ticks

It takes 2 to 3 years for ticks to develop from the egg stage to adults. All larval and adult stages of this parasite eat blood as their meals.

Spring and August and September are the high seasons for tick infestation. Adult female ticks prefer the cat's head and neck areas, whereas the larval stages favor the more hairless areas of the cat's body, like the edges of the ears, mouth, and eyes, and between the toes.

Symptoms

A few ticks on your cat won't hurt it more than a minor local inflammation, which will go away in just days.

Larger numbers of ticks cause severe itching, inflammation, and pus formation because of the animal's scratching, followed by secondary bacterial infections.

Causes

The most common tick that affects cats is Ixodes ricinus. *However, the type of ticks that might affect your cat depends on the geographical area you live in and on the type of terrain your cat is allowed to roam in.* Mites that live on hedgehogs and foxes affect cats as well.

Important: Humans may contract a virus through a tick bite. This infection may lead to encephalitis. Also, when you try to remove a tick with your fingers, the contact may transfer Borrelia (page 120) and cause disease.

Self-Help
The best tools for self-help are tick removers, or tick forceps, which you can buy at the veterinarian's office or at your pet store. Grasp the tick between the head and body of the tick with the forceps, turn the tool twice, and lift the tick right off the skin. Another method that also works quite well is the use of a highly alcoholic liquid. Dab a few drops on the tick. It will paralyze the tick and you can lift it off your cat's skin within a few minutes. It is best, however, to wait until the tick is dead before removing it.

Make sure that you do not touch the tick with your fingers. Instead, use a paper tissue, so as to avoid the chance of getting Borreliosis.

The other methods, like turning and pulling, or the use of oil to suffocate the tick, are not recommended because they cause the tick to excrete a substance that is highly inflammatory.

● Homeopathic Single Remedies
For the treatment of local inflammation with some pus formation administer Silica 12X for 7 days. It will calm the irritation quickly.

● Bach Flowers
Crab Apple is best for an internal and external cleansing program. For directions see page 84.

Combination Remedies
Traumeel ointment or Rescue cream are the most soothing and effective treatments of external inflammations.

Dosages for all remedies are listed on the inside front cover.

When to Get Professional Help
If your cat has a tick lodged in a critical area like the eyelid, or the edge of the eye, it might be necessary for a veterinarian to anesthetize the animal to remove the tick.

Prevention and Convalescent Care
Ticks are not a widespread problem for cats. Cats who have previously been heavily plagued by ticks should be fitted with a collar during the tick season. Quick and correct tick removal is the most important step you can perform.

Tapeworms

Tapeworms are made up of a head and a long chain of so-called proglottids. They live in the small intestine. The larval stages, also called fins, require intermediate hosts for their maturation. The cat can become the final host by eating an infected animal. Once the fins are ingested, they free themselves in the small intestine, where they take up residence and develop into mature tapeworms.

Symptoms
Tapeworms cause little or no symptoms in a cat. Kittens, on the other hand, react with clear symptoms such as a rough hair coat, lack of appetite,

7

weight loss, or even with enteritis, diarrhea, or vomiting.

Sexually mature tapeworms produce and expel large numbers of worm sections in the stool, each stuffed full with eggs. The tapeworm sections look like white rice as they stick to the hair in the anal region. There they cause itching, whereupon the cat tries to scratch and slide its little bottom along the floor.

Causes
The two major cat tapeworms are: Hydatigera taeniaeformis, the feline tapeworm, and the canine tapeworm, which parasitizes dogs *and* cats. Small rodents like rats and mice are the intermediate hosts of the feline tapeworm; fleas transport the canine tapeworm.

Neither of these tapeworms causes human disease.

Important: On rare occasions it is possible for cats to ingest a rodent that is infected with a fox tapeworm. In this way the cat could transmit tapeworm disease to humans.

Self-Help
Home remedies do not kill the worms, rather they change the intestinal environment in such a way that parasites do not care to live there anymore.

● Homeopathic Single Remedies
China 12X should be administered for 10 days. In addition, every worm treatment should be followed by an intestinal cleansing program which consists of two doses of Calcium carbonicum 30C, given 7 days apart.

● Bach Flowers
Use Crab Apple for internal cleansing.
For dosages see inside front cover.

When to Get Professional Help
When symptoms clearly indicate a potentially heavy worm infestation you should get professional help.

What Are the Treatment Options?
A stool exam will quickly determine the type and degree of worm infestation. Widely used antiparasitic medications will rid the cat of worms.

Prevention and Convalescent Care
Stool analysis should be performed twice every year. Treatment is needed only if there is evidence of worms.

Important: If you know that your cat eats mice occasionally, or if you are aware of fleas on your cat, you need to consider the chances for tapeworm infestation. Fleas and mice are the main transmitters of this disease to cats.

Roundworms

Roundworms are 2 to 4 in. (5 to 10 cm) long, white, and live in the small intestine of the cat, where they feed off the soft intestinal contents. The eggs and larval stages are ingested by the cat by licking or eating infected excrement, or by eating feral rodents, birds, or raw meat. Some of the larvae mature quickly in the wall of the intestine. Others migrate via the liver to the lung, where they are coughed up, only to be swallowed again, to begin their final maturation in the intestine.

Others may get encapsulated somewhere in the muscles of the cat, where they can remain intact for a long time. These encapsulated worms are of considerable importance in pregnant queens because pregnancy hormones are able to reactivate the enclosed worms. When the kittens are born the worms will be transmitted to them via the mother's milk.

Symptoms

Roundworm infestation in cats is quite widespread, but is seen without much associated disease.

Heavy worm infestation leads to rough fur, lack of appetite, weight loss, or vomiting and diarrhea. Worms may be visible in either the vomited material or in the stool. There are rare cases when heavy infestation may lead to constipation and organic deterioration, or where migrating larvae cause peritonitis or pneumonia. Newborn kittens may develop rickets, if they are burdened with severe worm infestation.

Cause

Toxocara felis is the roundworm that is specific for cats.

No matter where you live, there is a good chance that your cat will get infected with roundworm in its lifetime.

Toxocara leonina infects dogs predominantly, although it is able to infect cats.

Important: Humans are also susceptible to roundworms and their larvae. Children are especially at risk because they might be playing in a sandbox that has been used by cats as a litterbox.

Self-Help

● **Homeopathic Single Remedies**

Give Abrotanum 12X for 10 days. Follow with two administrations, one week apart, of Calcium carbonicum 30C, five globules each dose. This will change the intestinal milieu as needed.

● **Bach Flowers**

Symptoms	Treatment
General weakness	Olive
Evidence of endoparasites	Crab Apple

Dosages for all remedies are listed on the inside front cover.

When to Get Professional Help

In case of heavy worm infestation the veterinarian will use the appropriate worming medication to rid your cat of its disease.

Prevention and Convalescent Care

Get your cat's stool examined twice yearly (page 16). Always cook pork meats because raw meats may be infected.

The encapsulated larval stages of the roundworm are not affected by deworming medications. If a nursing mother is considered to be infected, the kittens must be treated against worms every 8 to 10 days as long as they are nursing. See the worm treatment chart on page 16.

Thorough hygiene of the litterbox and quick removal of the excreta are the most effective ways to prevent re-infections.

7

Infectious Diseases

Infectious diseases are caused by viruses, bacteria, or fungi. Infection occurs through contact, either directly or transported by droplets between cats. Indirect transmission is carried by objects, like food bowls, toys, blankets, or kitty baskets. Cats can also get infections from other animal or from humans. After a period of incubation (page 121), the cat will exhibit symptoms that are typical for the infectious agent.

Western medicine does not have effective treatments against viral infections, which gives homeopathic medicine a special place and meaning. Through its remedies the body is stimulated to increase its own defense mechanisms, and to heal itself. Recovery from viral infections carries, as a rule, a life-long immunity with it.

Bacterial infections in cats are, most commonly, the result of a primary viral infection, or the consequence of another underlying disease. With the discovery of antibiotics, Western medicine has developed effective treatments against bacterial infections. While an antibiotic fights only one specific bacterial infection, natural remedies rebalance the disturbed organism, thus strengthening the body to ward off other bacterial infections.

Fungal agents are found everywhere. Their spores are very resistant to environmental conditions, and they multiply quickly under favorable circumstances.

Systemic fungal infections affect entire organ systems, especially the intestines, the respiratory tract, and the central nervous system. These infections are very rare in cats.

On the other hand, mycotic skin infections are quite common in the cat, and they are transmissible to humans and other pets.

Feline Respiratory Complex (FRC)

This group of viral flu-like diseases is often accompanied by rhinitis, which is expressed by sneezing and by a runny nose.

Important: Nasal colds may be caused by allergic reactions, by irritations from mechanical obstructions, or by tumors.

Symptoms

Following an incubation period of 1 to 4 days, the cat starts to sneeze, and the nose is runny with a watery-thin discharge. Soon the eyes will get inflamed, and the animal turns into a tired, apathetic patient, who does not want to eat, and wants to be left alone.

Older, more resistant cats recover from the infection relatively quickly, but they continue to shed the virus, transmitting it to other cats.

Kittens and weak animals become severely ill. In addition to the other symptoms the eyes may develop keratitis or ulcerations. Stomatitis and pharyngitis develop frequently, and bacterial secondary infections superinfect the red, swollen, and severely inflamed mucosa. The condition is very painful. Two to three days later, the nasal discharge turns greenish-white, leaving caked, encrusted exudates in the nostrils. Salivation is increased, turns stringy, and appears hanging around the lips and mouth. As fever weakens the animal, it begins to cough, and turns pitifully apathetic. Finally, the lungs develop pneumonia, and severe coughing may follow.

Causes

The cat flu complex is caused by a group of viral infections, among them Calici virus, herpes virus, Rhinotracheitis virus, pneumonitis virus, and others. Secondary bacterial infections, especially of Chlamydial origin, may aggravate and severely complicate the disease.

Self-Help

If the eyes are affected by the disease, it as important to treat them topically (see page 34, "Conjunctivitis").

In order to relieve painfully encrusted nostrils you need to soak a little cotton in chamomile tea or in Calendula solution, and gently dab the crusty secretions until they can be wiped off.

● Homeopathic Single Remedies

Belladonna 12X is indicated for several days, three to six times daily, if the disease appears suddenly, if fever is present, and if the infection was caused either by a weather change or by transmission from another animal.

Pulsatilla 12X is indicated, if the nasal discharge has a yellow-greenish discoloration, if the animal refuses to drink, and if it shows distinct mood swings.

Allium cepa 6X, must be administered six times daily, if the nose is runny continuously, if the nostrils appear sore, and if it looks like the condition gets better outside, but worse indoors.

A specific nosode, derived from cat flu, may be administered in combination with the other treatments. It should be given at a 30C potency for 7 days at one dose daily.

● Bach Flowers

Symptoms	Treatment
Soiled, encrusted nose	Crab Apple
Weakened defenses	Centaury
Loss of strength to live	Hornbeam
Lack of ability to heal	Rescue Remedy

● Combination Remedies

Echinacea comp and Gripp-Heel are very effective for conditions of moderate severity. During the first few days you would need to administer one dose every 2 hours. If you alternate the two medications, your success rate will be higher. For the alleviation of pain under these circumstances give the animal Traumeel. Once the condition improves, you may reduce the dosage slowly until it is completely discontinued.

For dosages see inside front cover.

When to Get Professional Help

The animal should be treated by a veterinarian if the condition appears severe, if the animal is apathetic, and if your home treatment has not shown visible improvement.

What Are the Treatment Options?

A veterinary exam will include an antibiotic susceptibility test (page 120), and a blood analysis. In severe cases it will be unavoidable to treat the cat with an antibiotic, in order to prevent aggravating secondary bacterial infections.

Prevention and Convalescent Care

The cat flu complex is a common feline disease, which may, on occasion, be fatal. The best prevention is a consistent vaccination schedule.

8

Panleukopenia

This disease is known by terms such as feline distemper, Panleukopenia, and parvo-virus disease, and it is responsible for the majority of sudden kitten deaths. The mortality rate between the ages of 6 weeks to 4 months is about 90%.

A kitten that appears perfectly healthy in the evening could be dead by the following morning. This kind of sudden death is either due to poisoning or to parvo-virus infection.

Symptoms

The acute form of this disease has a short incubation period (page 121), which leads to a painful abdominal condition. The kitten won't let you touch its belly, it may vomit, and may have diarrhea. The vomited material is greenish-yellow, and stringy. The thin, or watery stool is foul smelling, and may be tinged with blood and mucus. In most cases there are ulcerated areas visible in the mucosa of the mouth, or small blisters surrounded by inflammation.

The animal appears miserable, is lethargic, and is in pain. Its hair is dull, and it seeks warm, quiet places from where it does not want to move. General weakness and dehydration set in quickly, and turn into a life-threatening condition. Usually the fever climbs soon, and the animal refuses food and water. As the condition progresses, the eyes appear sunken, and the conjunctiva turns pale. The latter is caused by the loss of white blood cells, for which the disease is called Panleukopenia. Unless therapy is started immediately, organic breakdown and dehydration soon lead to death.

If the disease develops the chronic form, the main symptom will be diarrhea. The degree of appetite varies, the hair coat stays dull, and the kitten continues to lose weight.

In general, it can be said that the disease is most destructive to the digestive tract and to the white blood cell system.

Causes

Parvo-virus is the infectious agent that is responsible for this disease. This virus is highly resistant to environmental factors, like heat and cold.

Self-Help

Cats who suffer from this disease require intensive care and attention. If the animal refuses food, it expresses its body's need for total rest. When you administer oral fluids (e.g., water or tea), add the homeopathic medication at the same time.

● Homeopathic Single Remedies

Wild Indigo is the specific remedy for this illness. Administer it in the form of Baptisia 6X over several days at one dose every 2 hours. In addition, administer four doses of Baptisia 30C on the first day, and two doses (mornings and evenings) on the following days.

Treat the kitten with Mercurius 12X if it shows heavy salivation, white deposits on the tongue, increased thirst, and blood-tinged, slimy stool.

China 6X is indicated in all cases where dehydration and general weakness are apparent. This medication is best administered in combination with other medications.

● Bach Flowers

Symptoms	Treatment
Apathy	Wild Rose
Response to viral multiplication	Crab Apple
Severe loss of vitality	Centaury
Acute and critical signs	Rescue
Severe inflammation	Holly

● **Combination Remedies**

Mercurius-Heel is indicated for cases where inflammatory disease generates pus. Use Diarrheel for cats with gastroenteritis and diarrhea. If you are dealing with a very weak animal you should give both medications on an alternating schedule for the first few days. Administer one dose every 2 hours, alternating three times on each day.

Dosages for all remedies are listed on the inside front cover.

When to Get Professional Help

A severely ill animal must be taken to a veterinarian without delay.

What Are the Treatment Options?

Dehydrated animals will receive intravenous electrolyte fluid before anything else. The veterinarian may increase the chances for recovery by injecting specific immune serum or by using an unspecific immune serum that assists the general buildup of immune defenses. If there is evidence, or increased risk for a secondary infection, this would be the right time to combine veterinary drug treatments with homeopathic remedies.

Serum analysis and an antibiotic susceptibility test (page 120) are usually necessary in order to assess the stage of the disease process.

Severely ill animals require intensive care for several days.

FIP

FIP is the abbreviated term for feline infectious peritonitis. This disease affects an increasing number of cats, and it is of major importance because of its high rate of mortality: 90 percent of affected cats will die. Many cats carry the virus without showing symptoms of disease. It looks clearly as if the virus awaits a second factor, like stress, parasitism, or territorial rivalries, before it will express itself in the form of disease. The virus can also be transmitted to the fetuses in a pregnant cat. The latter may explain the high number of viral carriers, and the reason why young cats who are affected by this disease have a very weak immune system to begin with.

The majority of cats that are affected by this disease are between the ages of 5 months and 6 years. The mouth is the tool for transmission of the virus. Symptoms develop after a long incubation period (page 121), ranging from weeks to months.

Symptoms

The first unspecific symptoms are fever, lack of appetite, and lethargy. The typical symptoms of peritonitis will not appear until later: Ascites and emaciation. At this stage the belly looks round and distended, while the ribs are showing on the chest. The abdominal cavity can accumulate as much as 1 quart (1 L) of peritoneal fluid.

In addition to this main expression of the disease, the lining tissues of other organs may be affected, e.g., those of the brain or of the chest cavity. There is also a so-called "dry" form of FIP, which is characterized by the absence of fluids, developing, instead, dry inflammatory deposits on the peritoneum.

Causes

The infectious agent is a corona virus.

Self-Help

Western medicine has no cure for FIP. Alternative medical treatments are worth trying, since homeopathic practice has reported cases of recovery.

8

● **Homeopathic Single Remedies**
A treatment course of 2 to 3 weeks with Arsen 12X is indicated in cases where ascites and other symptoms appear simultaneously. In addition it is necessary to administer Echinacea 4X, two to four times daily, in order to enhance the strength of the body's general defense abilities. If the abdomen of the animal is distended by the accumulation of the fluid, an additional treatment with Apocynum cannabium 4X is required at one daily dose for 8 to 10 days.

● **Bach Flowers**

Symptoms	Treatment
Internal toxins	Crab Apple
Loss of resistance	Centaury
Tiredness, exhaustion	Olive
Apathy	Wild Rose

● **Combination Remedies**
The most effective treatment for ascites (inflammatory fluid in the abdomen) is Apis-Homaccord, at a dose of five to seven drops, three times daily. In addition, two other homeopathic medicines are recommended: Arnica-Heel to increase the body's defenses and Galium-Heel to fight fluid accumulation and to produce unspecific defenses. Give five drops of each, three times daily, for several weeks.

Start the treatment with Apis-Homaccord. If the condition does not improve after 2 to 3 weeks, switch to Arnica-Heel or to Galium-Heel.

Dosages for all remedies are listed on the inside front cover.

What Are the Treatment Options?
A holistic veterinarian who specializes in homeopathic medicine will select the constitutional remedy that is indicated for this condition, and will administer it in high potency form.

Prevention and Convalescent Care
Regular immunizations are the best prevention (page 17).

Important: After a cat has died from FIP you should disinfect all bedding and contact areas to prevent other cats from getting infected.

Salmonellosis

Salmonella infection is transmitted by infected animals, e.g., birds and mice, by spoiled meats, or by soiled food bowls.

Symptoms
The gastrointestinal tract is the main target for this highly inflammatory disease. Diarrhea, frequently tinged with blood, leads to dehydration, and the cat becomes weak and lethargic. If the infection passes from the intestines into the blood, a septicemia (page 121) develops. This stage often ends in death, especially if the cat is young.

While a few cats get very ill when they are exposed to this infectious agent, most deal with it without any symptoms of disease. However, they do remain carriers, and shed the Salmonella bacteria, thus threatening other animals and humans with infection (anthropozoonosis, page 120).

Causes
Salmonella are bacteria that infect the digestive tract.

Self-Help
See "Diarrhea" on page 53 for home remedies.

Important: If salmonellosis is suspected, you, as cat owner, must be very cautious. Put on disposable gloves when you clean the litterbox or when you do any other cat cleaning chores.

Infections That Generate Pus

Streptococcal and Staphylococcal infections are the most common among the pus-producing bacteria.

Symptoms

Staphylococcal infections are at work when you observe pus-containing inflammatory areas on the skin, the ears, around the eyes, and also in the urinary tract, and the lungs, and wherever abscesses develop.

Streptococcal infections affect the mucosals of the head, the tonsils, and the lymph nodes of the head region. They are also found in inflammatory disease of the kidneys,and the pelvic area, where they are known to cause septicemia.

Self-Help

● **Homeopathic Single Remedies**

Abscesses, pus-containing inflammations, and other circumscribed areas should be treated with Hepar sulfuris 12X for 7 days. Once an abscess has broken open, Silicea 12X will finish the healing process.

Streptococcinum and Staphylococcinum are specific nosodes that are also effective against these bacterial infections.

● **Bach Flowers**

Crab Apple is indicated for heavily infected cases, while Centaury is more suitable to re-energize a weak cat.

● **Combination Remedies**

Use Belladonna-Homaccord for cats with severe infections, but Mercurius-Heel is better for inflammations with overt pus. Traumeel may be used in conjunction with other remedies, especially if there is pain.

For all dosages see inside front cover.

What are the Treatment Options?

For therapy references see "Abscesses" (page 68), "Inflammation of the Pharynx" (page 42), "Inflammatory Lesions of the Mouth" (page 39), and "Acute Nephritis" (page 59).

Infections With Coliform Bacteria

Infections with coliform bacteria are common in all organ systems. They may arise as specific diseases (e.g., mastitis), or they occur as a result of, or in conjunction with viral diseases, parasitism, or stress conditions. The eyes, ears, urinary tract, as well as nasal and pharyngeal passages are affected most frequently. The intestinal tract is a favored site for coli infections.

Symptoms

Primary coli infections cause septicemia in most cases (page 121). Secondary coli infections often aggravate the underlying viral disease, thus causing severe organic damage. This is what happens when a runny nose turns into a suppurative rhinitis (page 121).

Causes

These infections are caused by a variety of coliform bacteria, like Escherichia coli or Proteus.

8

Self-Help

Home remedies are indicated according to the type of symptoms: see, e.g., "Mastitis" (page 66), "Diarrhea" (page 53), and "Pneumonia" (page 47).

Prevention and Convalescent Care

Proceed according to symptoms, as for mastitis (page 66), enteritis (page 53), and pneumonia (page 47).

Fungal Skin Disorders

Symptoms

It takes about 2 to 4 weeks for a fungal infection to turn into symptomatic disease (dermatophytosis). The skin lesions appear as small round hairless areas that are slightly raised and scaly in the center. At the edge, there is an inflammatory ring, which is formed by the concentrically growing fungal spores. The spores (page 121) migrate into the hair follicles, creating hair loss. While the head is most often affected, the problem may be found on the body, the back, the limbs, or the tail.

The unrelenting itch of the infection causes the cats to scratch vehemently, which leads to aggravating secondary bacterial infections.

Causes

The main culprit is Microsporum canis, causing about 90% of all feline fungal infections. Microsporum gypseum, and a variety of Trichphyton forms are less frequently diagnosed.

Self-Help

The affected areas should be treated with Calendula solution [diluting 10 ml (¼ oz) of the mother tincture in 3 oz. (100 ml) of water].

Important: In order to prevent infection, you should wear disposable gloves when you treat the wounds of your cat.

● Homeopathic Single Remedies

Sepia 30C, administered every fifth day for several weeks, is the treatment of choice for female cats who suffer from dry scaly skin with hairless spots.

Use Natrium muriaticum 12X on dry, itchy, and scaly skin. Sulfur 12C is formulated for skin that smells poorly, appears dirty-red, and produces visible dander.

In highly resistant cases the use of nosodes, specifically Trichsporon and Microsporon, are indicated.

● Bach Flowers

Symptoms	Treatment
Skin infected and soiled	Crab Apple
Damaged skin	Rescue Remedy

Important: Crab Apple may be used externally and internally in cases of skin diseases. For external use dilute 10 drops of the internal formulation on 8 oz. (¼ L) water.

● Combination Remedies

Cutis comp. has had excellent results in the treatment of fungal infections. Administer daily ½ to 1 ampule in the drinking water, continuing for 2 to 3 weeks, or until the lesions have healed.

If the condition demands it, Schwef-Heel is highly effective. Give five drops, three times daily, for about 10 to 14 days.

Dosages for all remedies are listed on the inside front cover.

When to Get Professional Help

Fungal skin infections are usually very tough to treat. Consult a veterinarian before the condition worsens.

What Are the Treatment Options?

With the help of UV light from a Wood's lamp the veterinarian can diagnose the fungal infection. This allows the choice of the most suitable course of treatment aimed at cleansing the body internally to achieve healing.

Prevention and Convalescent Care

The risk of infection is very low if you pay attention to good nutrition, worm treatments, and general hygiene. Homeopathy and Bach Flowers are particularly suited for these infections because they are predominantly caused by constitutional problems.

Important: Cat owners, who are susceptible to fungi, should pay particular attention to matters of hygiene, because these infections are transmissible between cats and humans.

8

Practical Advice for Cat Owners

As a rule, cats are healthy, tough, resistant, and enduring animals. Only rarely do they get sick. Cats are more likely to get into trouble during their roaming excursions, injuring themselves or getting hit by cars. The next pages provide guidance for first aid, and for treatment in cases of emergency, poisoning, or burns. In addition, you will find useful tips on how to properly take care of a sick cat, how to prevent diseases, and how to apply correct bandages.

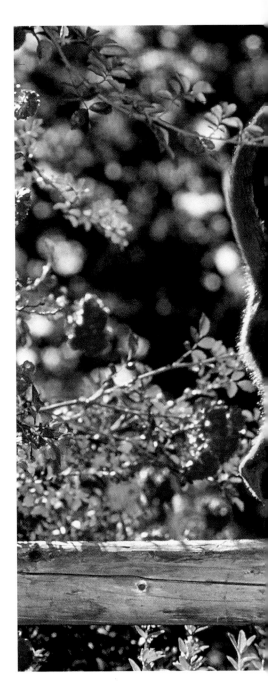

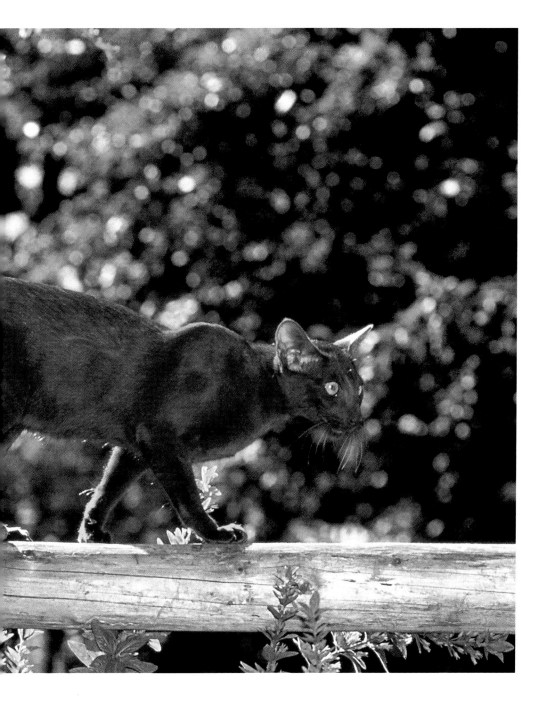

Practical Advice

A second person as a helper makes this task a lot easier. The normal temperature of cats lies between 100.5° and 102.5°F (38° and 39°C).

Preparing for a Doctor's Visit

Taking the Temperature

Taking the temperature of your cat should be the first thing you do when your cat gets sick. Digital thermometers with small tips are the easiest to handle.

Cover the tip of the thermometer with a little lubricating jelly. Lift the tail of your cat gently and slowly, while you insert the tip into the anal opening. The cat may stand or lie on its side for this procedure. Remember that cats do not like their tails lifted. Insert the tip approximately ¾ in. (2 cm) and hold it steady until the digital sound signals that the reading is done. While you are holding the thermometer for the reading you should talk to your cat in a reassuring voice, petting it until the ordeal is over.

Taking the Pulse

The best place to feel the pulse of a cat is on the inside of the thigh. You can do this while your cat stands or lies on its side. Apart from counting the number of beats per minute, you should also pay attention to the regularity and intensity of the pulse. The pulse rate is accelerated under normal circumstances, e.g., if you remove a cat from a cage. Therefore, do not count the pulse until you know that your animal has calmed down following any unusual happenings. The result is more reliable if you do the count at least twice in 5 minutes. Normal pulse rates range from 120 to 140 beats per minute.

Measuring the Rate of Breathing

The breathing frequency is measured by counting each inhalation and exhalation as one breath. To do this you can count the movement of the chest or of the belly. If a cat suffers from diseases of the lung, or of the circulatory system, breathing is accelerated. The same is true for conditions that cause abdominal pain, and for kidney problems. Normal breathing yields from 20 to 40 breaths per minute.

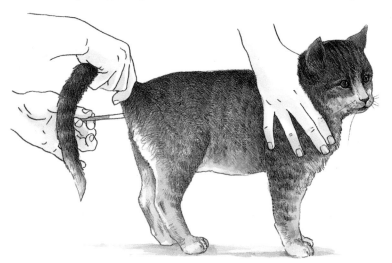

To measure the temperature, insert the tip of the thermometer approximately 1 in. (2 cm) horizontally into the anus. This procedure is much easier if you have a helper.

Important Symptoms to Watch For In Your Cat

Mouth
Saliva, tartar, loose teeth, inflammation, color

Nose Pad
Discharge, moisture, color

Eyes
Secretions, nictitating membrane, opaqueness, pupils, sensitivity to light, deposits

Ears
Discharge, irritated edges, itching, swelling, deposits in the ear canal

Anus
Caked deposits, color, parasites

Genitals
Discharge, color, swelling, reddening

Fur Coat
Hair loss, dander, parasites

Skin
Eczema, itching, parasites

Legs
Limping (which leg?), injuries, swelling

Paws
Nails, foot pads, spaces between the pads

How to Restrain Your Cat

Many cats resist as soon as one tries to examine them. Here are some pointers on proper restraint:

• For the chest-and-shoulder grip place both thumbs over the scruff of the neck, place the index fingers in front of the front legs, and cup the other fingers around the chest firmly but not too tightly.

• For the neck-and back grip grab the scruff of the neck firmly with your right hand, and place your left hand over the lower back area, while exerting gentle pressure downward with both hands.

• For the restraint of cats who vehemently refuse to allow cleaning or treatments of the eyes, ears, mouth, or face, it is necessary to wrap them into a blanket or towel, allowing only their head to emerge.

Important: Most treatment procedures are easier if you ask a second person to help hold the animal.

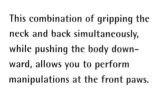

This combination of gripping the neck and back simultaneously, while pushing the body downward, allows you to perform manipulations at the front paws.

Practical Advice

Medicines

Most cats can be tricked into accepting tablets if you break them into little pieces and hide them inside a small meatball.

If your cat refuses to eat this, you need to grab the head from the back (see next page), as if you wanted to look inside the mouth, and place the tablet as far back on the tongue as you can. Then, you hold the mouth shut until the cat has swallowed. There are pill applicators that you can get at a pet supply store, which can make your task a lot easier.

Globules are best dissolved in a little water. Pull the liquid into a 2 cc plastic syringe (without the needle!), and instill it inside the cheek through the side of the mouth (see drawing next page). If you have a cat that requires daily injections, such as insulin, ask for instructions from your veterinarian.

Inhalation

Place the cat in a cage or basket, and cover three of the four sides with a towel. Heat water, and add chamomile or Kamillosan drops. Place the pot with the steaming infusion in front of the cage, and fan the steam into the cage toward the cat.

Important: Never treat your cat with medications that are formulated for humans. Never use expired medications, or medicine that does not appear to be in good condition.

Treating the Mouth Cavity

Hold the head of the cat from the back, placing your thumb and index fingers at the corners of the mouth. When you exert just a little pressure, the gums are pushed up against the teeth, and the cat will open its mouth. Use the index finger of the other hand to push the lower jaw down. Now you can inspect the inside of the mouth. A second person can help you hold the front legs.

Eye Treatments

Occasional runny eyes are wiped clean with a soft tissue, by wiping along the lower lid, from the outside toward the nose.

Severe eye inflammation or discharges must be treated with eye drops or ointments. Hold the

Medicine Cabinet for Cats

Medical supplies should be kept in an easily accessible area, where they are handy at a moment's notice.

✓ **Instruments and syringes**
   Digital thermometer, scissors, tweezers, tick forceps, nail cutter, disposable syringes (2 cc, 5 cc)

✓ **Medicines**
   Worming medication, lubricating jelly, ear cleaner, eye dropper and drops

✓ **Homeopathic remedies**
   Arnica, Belladonna, Hepar sulfuris, Mercurius, Nux vomica, Sulfur

✓ **Ointments**
   Calendula ointment, Traumeel ointment, Rescue cream

✓ **Bandaging supplies** (page 14)

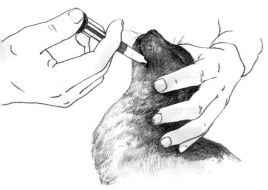

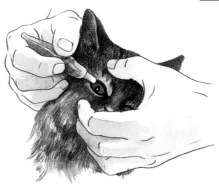

Administering medications into the mouth: The cat opens the mouth when you exert light pressure with thumb and index finger.

Administering eye medications: Always apply drops or ointments from the side, never from the top of the eyes.

head as in the drawing above, and place your thumb above the upper lid, using the index finger to gently pull the lower lid down. Open the eye only enough to drop about two to four drops into the lower lid. Allow the eye to close, and follow with gentle circular stroking to distribute the medication over the eye.

Important: If you suspect a foreign object in the eye, do not proceed with any topical treatment. Take the cat immediately to a veterinarian.

Ear Treatments

Infiltration of the ear with an ear cleanser precedes any medical treatment. Hold the outer ear upward, and introduce the bottle opening into the ear canal. Gently deliver the cleaning solution into the ear and massage the ear carefully to soften any dry crusty deposits on the inside. The cat will shake its head vigorously, and expel the loose particles. Use a tissue to clean the visible parts from the ear canal.

Administer medications in the same way.

Once the cat has shaken off most of the caked deposits you can follow on the second or third day by cleaning the ear gently with a cotton swab dipped in cleanser or medication.

Important: Eyes and ears should be examined carefully at least once every week!

Allopathic homeopathic remedies (page 120) must be stored separately from other medications. Never hold, store, or use homeopathic remedies simultaneously with any ethereal oils, camphor, Vick's Vapor-rub, or other similar strongly scented products.

Practical Advice

General Care and Maintenance Procedures

Nail Care

Torn nails, injured paw pads, and inflammation between the toes lead to painful limping and disablement of the paws.

The cat should lie on its side. Exert a little pressure on the front of the paw, and you will notice the nails protruding. Now you can examine the nails for length, and the paws and pads for inflammatory lesions between the toes and between the pads. Trim the nails only if the cat has not used them sufficiently on the scratch pad or outdoors. When you trim the nails of an outdoor cat you need to know that cut nails are no longer sharp, which could endanger a cat's life in situations when the animal needs to escape. Use a nail trimmer to cut the nails, and be careful not to injure the blood vessel that runs along the center of the nail.

Taking Care of the Fur Coat

Cats are devoted to grooming their fur until it is shiny and clean. Dull, or rough hair conditions are sure signs that your cat is ill. A cat's tongue is perfectly designed for cleaning, being provided with a rough surface, and with several papillae. As a rule, cats will either eliminate the hair that is swallowed during grooming, or, if too much is accumulated, they might regurgitate it from the stomach. Long-haired cats, as well as semi-long-haired cats must be brushed thoroughly every day. Without daily fur care these cats would suffer from gastritis or from matted hair. Combing and brushing your cat should become a welcome ritual, not a hateful necessity.

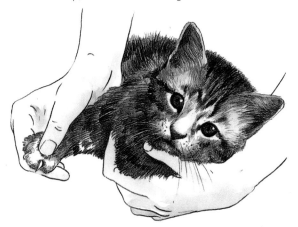

Light pressure on the front of the paw causes the nails to protrude. Now you can check whether they are too long.

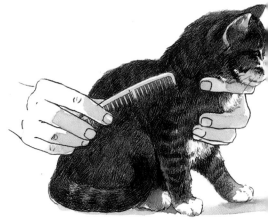

While you are combing your cat, make sure you follow the direction of the hair growth.

General Health Care Methods

Always pet your cat before you begin combing or brushing. Be sure to comb in the direction of natural hair growth, i.e., from the head toward the tail. Use your fingers to pull apart small knots and mats, then follow with a wide-toothed comb. Heavily matted hair should be cut away with a hair trimming knife. Should you encounter large areas of matting that are painful to remove, you should take the animal to a veterinarian to have the removal done under anesthesia. Remember to check your cat for any abnormal skin changes, parasites, or injuries.

Brushing follows after the combing. The brush removes loose hairs and smoothes the fur. Pay close attention to the belly, the insides of the thighs, and to the hairs between the paw pads and toes.

Shorthair cats, like Abyssinians, Siamese, British Shorthairs, and Domestic Shorthairs, need to be combed and brushed only during the shedding season.

Bathing Your Cat

Cats need to be bathed if they are heavily soiled, and if they are infested with parasites. Most cats detest bathing, and you should prepare everything you need before the bath, in order to absolve the ordeal quickly. Get a plastic pitcher, the shampoo or dip, and a pre-warmed towel ready, before you get the cat.

Fill one half of a plastic tub with warm water, at about 95°F (35°C). Place the cat carefully into the water, while you hold its front legs, and use the other hand for shampooing and rinsing.

Dry the cat thoroughly in the pre-warmed towel, and carry the animal into a warm room, where it can remain until the fur is dry.

Important: Do not soak the head, and be careful not to get shampoo in the eyes or ears!

Taking Care of the Anal and Genital Areas

Caked deposits in the anal area are easily removed with a moist paper towel. If matted hair is stubbornly tangled, use a pair of scissors, and cut the clumps carefully away. Healthy cats keep their anal region meticulously clean. When you notice caked anal deposits, you should consider the possibility that your cat is suffering from some type of digestive tract disorder.

Checking the condition of the genital area is especially important when you are dealing with a pregnant or nursing queen. Any discharge may be a signal of disease, and you should get veterinary help immediately.

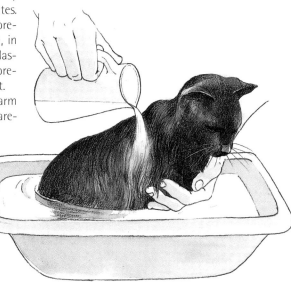

Because cats dislike bathing, it is a good idea to hold the front paws of your cat during this ordeal.

Practical Advice

Feeding Sick Cats

In addition to intensive care, sick cats need the appropriate nutrition. If your cat refuses food, this may unburden the digestive tract. Allow the cat to fast, and offer it fresh water, or tea, if diarrhea is present. After about 2 days the body has usually detoxified its system, and the animal should start to show interest in food. Offer your cat a favorite snack or food, like meat, fish, or a special canned food.

The cat's appetite needs to be restored as quickly as possible to prevent secondary complications (e.g., hepatic lipidosis). Therefore, if the sick cat continues fasting after 3 days, you will need to force-feed the animal in order to stimulate the appetite and to maintain its physical strength. One of the most favored methods is to form small meatballs, and place them in the cat's mouth; warming the meatball will increase the cat's desire for food. Or, you can stimulate the appetite by dissolving 1 teaspoon of fructose in 250 ml water, and then drip some of this solution into the cat's mouth. Under the direction of a veterinarian you may also administer bovine serum as an appetite enhancer. To administer these liquids, hold the cat gently by the scuff of the neck, and use a spoon to dribble the fluids into the side of the mouth. You can do the same thing with a disposable syringe (without a needle!).

Important: Do not administer a fructose solution if your cat suffers from an intestinal disorder with diarrhea. For the prevention of dehydration you need to get an electrolyte solution from the veterinarian.

Diets

There are a number of reasons why cats might need to be fed special diets: Reduce weight, relieve a chronically sick organ system, or to improve metabolic disorders. Any specific combination of food components can be considered a "diet."

Today you can find commercially available diets for just about any disorder. If you want to prepare special diets for your cat at home, you may follow the suggestions listed below.

Weight Loss Diet

A weight loss diet should have reduced amounts of fat and protein. Instead, it should contain more bulk, like rice and vegetables.

Do not try to place your cat on a zero-calorie diet, as you would a dog. Cats will find a way to beg for food at your neighbors.

Sample Weight Loss Diets
100 g cooked liver
60 g cooked, unsalted rice
2 tbsp. cooked vegetables
1 tsp. calcium carbonate
1 tbsp. cottage cheese

Diet for Kidney Failure
50 g cooked liver
1 to 2 hard boiled eggs
120 g cooked unsalted rice
10 g animal fat
½ tsp. calcium carbonate

Diet for Kidney Stones
120 g cooked beef
30 g cooked beef liver
45 g cooked unsalted rice
½ tsp. calcium carbonate
½ tsp. corn oil or thistle oil

If a cat refuses to eat for more than 2 days it is time for force-feeding. A spoon serves this purpose quite well.

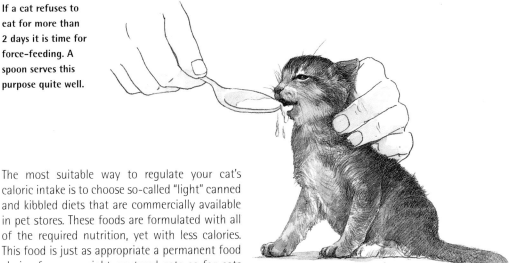

The most suitable way to regulate your cat's caloric intake is to choose so-called "light" canned and kibbled diets that are commercially available in pet stores. These foods are formulated with all of the required nutrition, yet with less calories. This food is just as appropriate a permanent food choice for overweight neutered cats as for cats that have too little exercise. There are a number of manufacturers, like Hills, Iams, and Eukanuba, who specialize in this type of diet.

Kidney Diet

A kidney diet is formulated with the goal to unburden kidney functions during the course of kidney disease. Protein and phosphorus content must be reduced, while calcium and vitamin A must be enriched. In addition, you must make sure that the cat takes in lots of fluids.

A veterinarian has to determine whether or not a kidney disorder can be regulated by a diet.

Liver Diet

In the case of liver disorders the protein in the food should be derived from fish, dairy products, cottage cheese, or tofu. Mix any of these ingredients with cooked rice; never with wild rice, however. In addition, add vitamins and minerals to formulate an easily digestible, nutritious meal.

Diet for Digestive Tract Disorders

A cat with gastrointestinal problems is first placed on 2 days of fasting, and then fed cottage cheese and mashed potatoes. Prepare the potatoes with water, not milk. Subsequently, the animal may eat small portions of chicken, beef, venison, as well as cooked liver, rice, and hard-boiled eggs.

Sufficient fluid intake is important at this time, because diarrhea and vomiting cause heavy loss of body fluids.

Important: Regardless of the type of diet, the minimum protein requirement of 5 g for each 5 kg of body weight must be met. Most diets are best fed on a two meals per day schedule. In cases of kidney or liver diseases this may have to be followed for the rest of the cat's life.

practical Advice

Accidents

Every feline life has some type of emergency in store, be it an accident, a fall from a window, or a poisoning. The right time to prepare for what to do in these emergencies is a quiet hour when you have time to think and to plan.

Accident

When a cat gets hit by a car, you need to manage the traffic situation first. Then, place the animal gently on a blanket, a cloth, or a coat, and transport it to a quiet location. Perform a quick exam, measuring the pulse (page 100), counting the breaths (page 100), and verifying the pinch reflexes (by pinching the outer ear or by touching the top of the eyelids). If you get no reaction, the cat is unconscious.

If you are not alone, ask someone to call the closest veterinary emergency clinic, and make arrangements to take the animal there as fast as possible. Arnica 12X should be administered, if it is available (see box at right). Then, reexamine the cat for injuries, bleeding, fractures, etc. Stop any heavy bleeding by tying a bandage as described on page 113.

Do not try to bandage or correct a broken leg or any open fracture wound. The latter would make things worse, and you would cause the cat unnecessary pain.

With the help of a second person try to place the cat into a cage or carton, with its broken limb on the top. Cover the animal to provide warmth. Administer a second dose of Arnica 12X before you leave for the veterinary clinic.

Important: Never leave an injured cat alone. Stroke the animal gently, and talk in a reassuring voice.

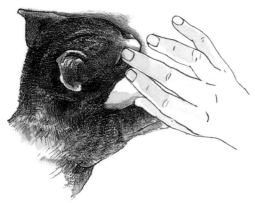

Eyelid reflex: Only unconscious cats fail to react to a light touch on the lid.

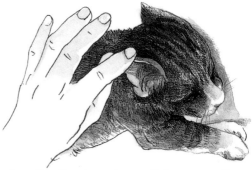

Ear reflex: Conscious cats move their ears as a reflex, when they are touched lightly.

Following an accident a cat should be placed on its right side in order to alleviate pressure on the heart.

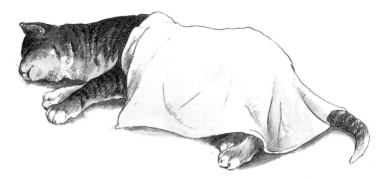

Unconsciousness

An unconscious cat fails to respond with reflexes. Pry the mouth open immediately, and check for any food particles. Carefully pull the tongue out to the side to make sure that the air passages are clear. Place the animal on its right side, and keep the head slightly elevated. Administer Arnica in the highest potency you have at home. Place the globules directly on the mucosa of the mouth, or dissolve them in water, and apply them drop by drop on the tongue.

Injuries From Falling

Falls from windows and balconies most frequently cause contusions, sprains, and fractures. Always have a veterinarian check the cat after this type of accident. Cover the cat, and administer Arnica 12X, or Rescue Remedy (see box at right), and go to the clinic immediately.

For self-help with injuries see page 78 and with fractures see page 80.

Bite, Stab, and Shot Wounds

These three injuries can be treated similarly.

First, give your cat Arnica 12X, or Rescue Remedy three times each day, for several days, even if the animal is scheduled for surgery.

Should an abscess develop, change the treatment to Hepar sulfuris 12X. If the abscess breaks open, or if a fistula develops, administer Silicea 12X. All of these medications are given at the dose of one tablet or three to five globules two to three times daily.

Important: If the injury was caused by a shot, you must take the cat to a veterinarian immediately. An x-ray will determine whether a bullet is lodged in the body, and if so, it must be removed surgically. If the shot entered a body cavity, surgical support is required immediately.

Emergency Remedies

Following any accident treat a cat with two to five globules of Arnica 12X every 15 minutes; or you can use two drops of Bach Flower's Rescue Remedy. If you do not have a 12X potentized formulation, you can use any other concentration.

Another choice is to administer both medications, by alternating them every 15 minutes.

Practical Advice

Poisoning

Cats do not get poisoned frequently because they are, in general, quite careful in their approach to unfamiliar substances, and they vomit readily. A list of typical symptoms that accompany poisoning accidents is shown on the right.

Cats like to chew on grass in order to regurgitate hairballs, or to regulate an uneasy stomach feeling. This habit gets cats into trouble, if they chew on poisonous grass. Offer your cat its own grass plants, like wheatgrass, papyrus, green lillies, etc.

Paints, lacquers, and chemicals of all sorts mat and soil your cat's hair, and, worse, they threaten your pet's life. Cats ingest the poison by licking the substances right off their coat.

How to Treat Poisoned Cats

Nux vomica C30 is the choice treatment for all types of poisonings. On the first day administer five globules three times, then, follow from the second day on with five globules twice daily. You can give the globules directly into the mouth, or dissolved in water.

If the hair is matted or caked with paint or lacquer, cut it away. Sections that cannot be cut should be cleaned thoroughly with solvents, and rinsed with much water. You then need to bathe the cat (page 105). Wrap the animal in a towel or blanket so that it cannot lick any remaining spots of the offending substance.

Drowning

Most cats that are pulled out of the water are unconscious, and have water in their lungs. Hold the cat by the hind legs, and stroke the chest with light pressure toward the head. This will move some of the water from the lungs outward. Repeat this procedure several times, resting for 10 to 20 seconds between each attempt.

If heart and lungs do not respond quickly, you will need to perform artificial respiration.

Place the cat on its right side to perform heart massage. Place your right hand behind the cat's left front leg and shoulder blade, and exert pressure on the chest, rhythmically pushing down and relaxing. Each massage action should last about 1 to 2 seconds.

If you have to perform artificial resuscitation, you need one person to hold the head up, while

Typical Symptoms of Poisoning

✔ **Salivation, Vomiting, Diarrhea**
Rat poison, disinfection agents, phenols

✔ **Bleeding**
Rat poison

✔ **Imbalance**
Analgesics, such as aspirin, antifreeze chemicals

✔ **Muscular tremor, Spasms, Contractions, Loss of consciousness**
Insecticides, pesticides, antifreeze

✔ **Hypothermia**
Pupils dilated, narrowed

✔ **Pale conjunctiva**
Blood poisoning

✔ **Yellow, discolored conjunctiva**
Liver disease (jaundice)

This is the right way to hold a cat that was about to drown. Use the other hand to stroke the chest toward the head to remove water from the lungs.

you grab the head with both hands, cover the cat's mouth and nose with your mouth and begin blowing for about 3 to 4 seconds at a time, until the chest starts to move visibly. Pause for an equal 3 to 4 seconds before each new firm blow. Continue these alternating actions for 3 to 4 minutes. By then, breathing has to be reestablished.

If you are dealing with an apparently cold, lifeless cat, and you have medicines available, place a few drops of Camphora 30X on the animal's tongue. On the other hand when the cat starts to make long drawn snoring sounds as the breathing begins, administer Opium 30C.

Suffocating

If you hear the cat coughing and gagging at the same time, lack of oxygen soon follows. Should you be aware that a foreign body is lodged in the throat, act immediately. If a second person is present, have one person hold the cat firmly, while you pry open the mouth, and, using a flashlight, inspect the back of the throat. If you see the object, grab it with a pair of tweezers, and pull it

out. Do not try to grab it with your fingers because the panicking cat will bite you. As soon as you are through with the ordeal give the cat three globules of Arnica 12X.

If you cannot remove the foreign body, or do not know the cause of the breathing impairment, take your cat immediately to an emergency clinic.

Burns

Burn injuries, whether with blister formation or without, must be cooled immediately. You can either dab the burned area gently with cold water, or place ice cubes in a cloth bag on the wounds. An even better method is to use water and vinegar, mixed 1:1, in which you soak a cloth, and use it to gently cover the affected area. Renew the cloth after a while because the calming effect of the vinegar evaporates with time.

On the following day begin the application of Rescue Cream on the damaged tissue areas. Cantharis 12X, at one dose, two to three times daily, is especially effective when the burn has caused blisters.

A poisoned or traumatized cat should be taken to a veterinary hospital immediately. If this is not possible, you should act according to emergency instructions from a veterinarian.

practical Advice

Bandages and Restraint

The wounds which usually require bandages are leg wounds and bites somewhere on the body surface, mainly along the chest or belly.

It is easier to bandage an animal if a second person helps you hold the cat. This way you can concentrate unhurriedly on treating the injury with ointments and bandages. A bandage must be wrapped firmly, but not so firmly that blood circulation is interrupted and the injured area swells.

Bandaging an Injured Paw or Leg
First, you need to clean the wound carefully and thoroughly, dabbing it dry with a clean tissue. The next layer is a Fucidine-gauze pad, which prevents the bandage from sticking to the wound. Once the

bandage has been changed repeatedly, you replace the Fucidine-gauze with wound balm. Place small pieces of gauze or cotton between the foot pads and the toes in order to prevent inter-digital inflammation.

The next layer consists of cotton or cellulose bandage materials, which is held in place over the paw or leg with a moderately firm placement of a gauze bandage. Be sure to cover the paw from all sides.

Use tape on the top and bottom of the bandage, making sure that the fur sticks to the tape to hold it in place, then wrap a second piece of tape criss-cross along the leg or foot, including front, back, and bottom.

Three or four pieces of tape will enable you to position the bandage firmly, and keep it attached to the fur, so that it won't move away from the wound.

Important: If you find a bandage stuck to the wound, moisten it with chamomile tea, and then lift it off gently with a pair of scissors.

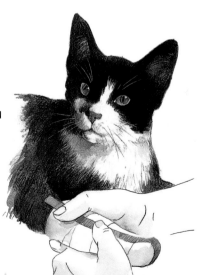

Bandages on paws or legs must be fixed with tape to the cat's fur to prevent them from slipping off the limbs.

Bandaging Materials
- Traumeel, or Calendula ointment, Rescue cream
- Fucidine gauze
- Cotton
- Sterile compresses
- Gauze bandages
- 2 elastic bandages
- Bandage tape
- Scissors with dull points
- Triangular cloth, safety pins, if available

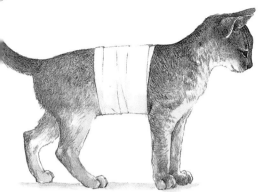

Wounds in the area of the chest or belly should be bandaged with a wide gauze bandage.

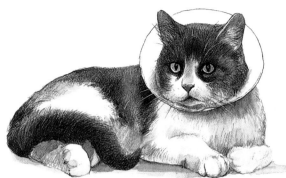

Elizabethan collars prevent cats from tearing off their bandages.

Chest Bandage

Injuries in the area of the chest should, at first, be protected by a healing ointment and bandage. As soon as healing has begun, the wound will progress better if left uncovered, and exposed to the air.

Dab a thin layer of Calendula ointment over the wound, and cover it with gauze, followed by some cotton for impact protection. Cover the area with a wide gauze bandage. On top of this you may follow with an elastic bandage, or you can use a triangular piece of cloth, a handkerchief, or any strips of fabric, like cotton sheets. If the wound appears extensive, you should take the cat to a veterinarian in case stitches are necessary.

How to Stop Bleeding Wounds

First, place a compress directly on top of the bleeding wound, and continue by wrapping a bandage firmly over it to exert pressure on the bleeding vessel. Then, take the animal without delay to a veterinarian.

After about 30 minutes you should loosen the bandage for a moment, in order to allow circulation to function temporarily.

Restraint

Many cats will try to chew off their bandages, as soon as you have finished putting them on. These patients need to be fitted with an Elizabethan collar, which is a plastic funnel that prevents the cat from reaching the bandage with its teeth. Another type of restraint is placing the cat in a cage following a bone fracture. This "forced rest" procedure ensures better, and quicker healing of the bones.

114

Index of Home Remedies

The following is a list of all homeopathic single remedies, combination remedies, and Bach Flowers, which are referred to in this book. Single remedy references contain details about *constitutional remedies (CR)*. Under "Indications" you will find the symptoms that are characteristic for the substance, and which require special attention for the choice of treatment.

Homeopathic Single Remedies

Unless otherwise noted in the text, all single remedies are available at the given potencies, either in the form of tablets (20 g), or in the form of globules (10 g).

Abrotanum
Indication: Endoparasites

Aconitum
A. napellus
Indication: Sudden health problems following exposure to cold air; fever during initial stage; strong fears

Aethusa
Indication: Vomiting sour milk

Allium cepa
Indication: Irritating nasal cold

Apis
A. mellifica
Indication: Severe redness, swelling, heat, pain, sensitivity to touch (such as from a bee sting), edema, relief with cool compresses

Apocynum cannabium
Indication: Abdominal ascitis

Arnica
A. montana
Indication: All injuries, e.g., punch, hit, squeeze, tear, wounds; soft tissue wounds with hematoma; before and after surgeries to prevent shock

Arsenicum album
Indication: Exhaustion with restlessness and fear; cold body and limbs; poisoning from spoiled meats; aggravation of a condition after midnight (1 to 3 A.M.); strong thirst, drinks often but small quantities; diarrhea with blood; exhaustion; improvement with warmth and with warm fluids

Baptisia
Indication: Panleukopenia

Belladonna
Indication: Sudden onset of febrile illnesses, with reddening and heat in the area of the head; cold limbs; high fever

Berberis
B. vulgaris
Indication: Kidney and bladder problems, urinary calculi

Borax
Sodium borate
Indication: Aphts, ulcers of the mouth

Bryonia
B. alba
Indication: Bronchitis, pneumonia, pleurisy; pain relief through pressure on the affected side (i.e., a cat with a left-sided bronchitis favors lying on the left side); improvement through rest, aggravation through any mobility; rheumatic pain

Calcium carbonicum (CR)
Indication: Most effective in kittens with problems during their growth phase; bone calluses; enlargement of the lymph nodes and glands; chronic catarrh; sensitivity to cold; large, white, and paste-like stools; diarrhea with milk intolerance (kittens)

Calcium phosphoricum
Calcarea phosphorica
Indication: Growth problems, bone fractures

Calendula
C. officinalis
Indication: Injuries, wounds, eye lesions

Cantharis
Indication: Kidney and bladder inflammations with strong urge to urinate

China (also Chinchona)
China officinalis
Indication: General weakness following loss of body fluids, or after severe illness

Chionanthus
Indication: Diabetes; pancreatitis

Conium
C. maculatum
Indication: Hard ulcers

Drosera
Indication: General strengthening of the defense mechanism

Euphrasia
Indication: Inflammations of the eyes:
Available as tablets (20 g), globules (10 g), drops of the mother tincture for external use (20 ml)

Ferrum
Indication: Anemia

Graphites (CR)
Indication: Overweight, fat, and bulky cats with constipation, skin disorders, eczema (mainly in the joint areas and behind the ears), and thick, honey-like exudates; thickened, brittle claws; sensitive to cold

Haronga
Indication: Pancreatitis

Hepar sulfuris
Indication: All types of suppurative inflammation (up to a potency of 6X pus will be expelled through the surface; higher potencies cause the pus to be resorbed through internal functions); strong sensitivity to cold (see Silicea); condition worsens under the slightest exposure to draft, cold, or dry wind; relief through warmth (seeks the heater, sun); excretions smell like ripe cheese

Hypericum
Indication: Nerve injuries and pressure injuries

Ignatia
Indication: Cats who are nervous, irritable, trembling, easily excitable, with mood changes, contrary behaviors; medication for sadness and worries (Natrium muriaticum, Pulsatilla)

Ipecacuanha
Indication: Cough with vomiting, difficulties in breathing

Iris versicolor
Indication: Pancreatitis

Jodum
Indication: Emaciation despite hunger and food intake; pancreatitis

Lachesis
Indication: Severe inflammation, predominantly of the left side

Lycopodium (CR)
Indication: Diseases of the digestive system and urinary tract; bloating after small amounts of food intake; hepatitis; emaciation despite voracious eating; hungry at night; frequent urination at night; impotence; brown spots on the skin of the belly; symptoms predominantly on the right side; problems move from right to left; conditions worsen between 4 and 8 P.M.

Mercurius (CR)
Indication: Severe inflammation of the ears, mouth, eyes, gastrointestinal tract; exudates are thick, yellow, and foul smelling (ear), or burning (eyes); tongue is swollen with teeth imprints, and white deposits (mouth); edematous gingivitis with bad mouth odors, and salivation; aphts in the oral mucosa; weakness and trembling of the limbs; diarrhea with foam and blood

Natrium muriaticum (CR)
Indication: Cats become severely emaciated; loss of vitality expressed by weakness and exhaustion; results of experienced fears and sadness; shyness, retreating; distrust toward strangers; dry, itchy, scaly skin eczema; Nat. mur. cats do not forget negative experiences, no matter how long ago they occurred

Natrium sulfuricum
Indication: Liver disorders; most important remedy for head injuries

Nux vomica (CR)
Indication: Spastic conditions of the digestive tract (colic, constipation, urge to defecate); hypersensitivity of the nervous system; hypersensitivity to noise, odors, light; colds from wind; back pain; hernias (with complications)

Opium
Indication: Intestinal spasms with pain, colic

Phosphorus (CR)
Indication: The phosphorus cat is tall, slim, with a narrow chest, affectionate, playful, small-boned, seeking company; tends to have bleeding that is hard to stop (e.g., from the nose, or after tooth extraction); prefers cold water; laryngitis, bronchitis, pneumonitis with cough, and impeded breathing; lying on the left side aggravates the condition; easily scared

Phytolacca
Indication: Mastitis, tumors of the mammary glands

Podophyllum
Indication: Diarrhea, which is eliminated under much pressure

Pulsatilla (CR)
Noteworthy is the changing nature of the symptoms (e.g., stool changes from too soft to too hard); frequently these are female cats, affectionate, a little moody; prefer cool rooms or outdoors; no signs of thirst; ocular and nasal secretions are thick, greenish-yellow, nonirritating

Rhus toxicodendron
Indication: Sprains, tears, torsion of the limbs or joints; moving around betters the condition; restlessness; wants cold milk (see phosphorus); pustular acne that itches strongly

Sepia (CR)
Indication: Remedy predominantly for female cats; during
heat the cat bites the approaching
tomcat; tends to abort fetuses;
metritis (important remedy for
uterine conditions); indifference
to own offspring; (see Lycopodium); likes to move about; prefers
being single cat

Silicea
Indication: Lack of vitality; cold
extremities; seeking warmth; emaciated kittens with delayed growth
and bloated bellies; abscesses, fis-
tulas, and pus-containing wounds,
which have already opened (see
Hepar sulfuris); glandular swelling
(see Calcium carbonicum); post-
vaccination disorders; digital
inflammation; fear of needles and
syringes

Spongia
Indication: Cough

Staphisagria
Indication: Cough

Sulfur (CR)
Indication: Highest recommended
skin medication; rough, dull hair
with dander; strong itching, even
without eruptions; foul-smelling
exudates; dry eczema; body orifices red (nostrils, eyes, anus,
vulva); diarrhea mornings; cat
wakes frequently ("cat napping"),
particularly between 3 and 5 A.M.;
bathing is not tolerated. Sulfur
30C is especially effective when
other medications failed, and
after a course of antibiotics, to
strengthen the overall condition

Symphytum
Indication: Bone fractures

Thuja
Indication: Warts, knots

Combination Remedies

Albumoheel (Heel)
Ingredients: Apis, Phos., Ign.,
Verat., Ter., a/o.
Indication: Kidney and bladder
disorders
Available as: Tablets (50 pcs.)

Angin-Heel (Heel)
Ingredients: Merc., Apis, Phyt.,
Arn., Hep., a/o.
Indication: Tonsillitis, pharyngitis
Available as: Tablets (50 pcs.)

Apis-Homaccord (Heel)
Ingredients: Apis, Ant-t., Scilla,
Indication: Edema, urine retention
with acute nephritis
Available as: Tablets (50 pcs.)

Arnica-Heel (Heel)
Ingredients: Arn., Bry., Colch.,
Echi., Bapt., a/o
Indication: Inflammation, or
injuries, localized or systemic
Available as: Drops [1 oz. (30 ml)]

Belladonna-Homaccord (Heel)
Ingredients: Bell., Echi.,
Indication: Severe inflammation,
localized or generalized
Available as: Drops [1 oz. (30 ml)],
ampules (5 pcs., 1.1 ml ea.)

Berberis-Homaccord (Heel)
Ingredients: Berb., Coloc., Verat.,
Indication: Inflammation of the
urinary tract
Available as: Drops [1 oz. (30 ml)],
ampules (5 pcs. 1.1ml ea.)

Bryaconeel (Heel)
Ingredients: Bry., Acon., Phos.,
Indication: Respiratory infections
Available as: Tablets (50 pcs.)

Calcoheel (Heel)
Ingredients: Calc., Dulc., cham.,
carb. veg.
Indication: Disorders of the mineral metabolism; glandular
swelling
Available as: Tablets (50 pcs.)

Calendumed (Heel)
Ingredients: Calendula
Indication: External for injuries
Available as: Ointment [2 oz. (50
g)], cream [2 oz. (50 g)]

Cantaris compositum (Heel)
Ingredients: Canth., Merc., Hep., a/o
Indication: Nephritis and/or
cystitis
Available as: Ampules (4 pcs.,
2.2 ml ea.)

Carcinomium compositum (Heel)
Ingredients: Carc., Sulf., Puls., a/o
Indication: Strengthening of the
immune system for cancer
Available as: Ampules (2 pcs.,
2.2 ml ea.)

Cardiacum (Heel)
Ingredients: Arn., Cact., Gels.,
Spig., Sulf., a/o
Indication: Cardiovascular weakness
Available as: Tablets (50 pcs.)

Chelidonium-Homaccord (Heel)
Ingredients: Chel., Bell., a/o
Indication : Diseases of the liver
and gallbladder
Available as: Drops [1 oz. (30 ml)],
ampules (5 pcs., 1.1 ml ea.)

China-Homaccord (Heel)
Ingredients: China, Sepia
Indication: Critical weakness
following severe illness
Available as: Drops [1 oz. (30 ml)],
ampules (5 pcs., 1.1 ml ea.)

Cinnamomum-Homaccord N (Heel)
Ingredients: Cinna., Ham., Mill.
Indication: Bleeding
Available as: Drops [1 oz. (30 ml)],
ampules (5 pcs. 1.1 ml ea.)

Crataegus-Heel (Heel)
Ingredients: Crataegus
Indication: Cardiovascular
weakness
Available as: Drops [1 oz. (30 ml)]

Cutis compositum (Heel)
Ingredients: Ign., Merc., Sulf.,
Thuja, organ extracts, a/o
Indication: Skin disorders
Available as: Ampules (4 pcs., 2.2
ml ea.)

Diarrheel (Heel)
Ingredients: Carb. m., Arg. n.,
Colch., Coloc., Podo., a/o
Indication: Diarrhea, gastroenteritis
Available as: Tablets (30 pcs.)

Duodenoheel (Heel)
Ingredients: Anac., Arg.-n., Ip.,
Jod., Lach., a/o
Indication: Enteritis
Available as: Tablets (50 pcs.)

Dysenteral (Wera Vet)
Ingredients: Ars., Rheum., Podo.
Indication: Diarrhea
Available as: Drops (20 ml)

Echinacea compositum S (Heel)
Ingredients: Echi., Acon., Bapt.,
Lach., Puls., a/o
Indication: Increase of body's
defenses during inflammatory
conditions
Available as: Ampules (4 pcs.,
2.2 ml ea.)

Febrisal (Wera Vet)
Ingredients: Acon., Lach., Echi.,
Indication: For acute fever
conditions
Available as: Drops (20 ml)

Ferrum-Homaccord (Heel)
Ingredients: Ferr., Ferr.-p., Ferr.-s.,
a/o
Indication: Iron deficiency
Available as: Drops [1 oz. (30 ml)],
ampules (5 pcs. 1.1 ea.)

Gastricumeel (Heel)
Ingredients: Arg.-n., Puls., Nux v.,
Carb. v., a/o
Indication: Gastritis
Available as: Tablets (50 pcs.)

Graphites-Homaccord (Heel)
Ingredients: Graph., Calc.
Indication: Disposition for obesity;
skin disorders
Available as: Drops [1 oz. (30 ml)],
ampules (5 pcs., 1.1 ml ea.)

Gripp-Heel
Ingredients: Acon., Bry., Lach.,
Eup.-per., Phos.
Indication: Flu-like diseases;
pharyngitis
Available as: Tablets (50 pcs.),
ampules (5 pcs., 1.1 ml ea.)

Heelax (Heel)
Ingredients: Aloe, Rheum., Coloc.,
Nux v., Bry.
Indication: Constipation
Available as: Pills (30 pcs.)

Hepeel (Heel)
Ingredients: Lyc., Chel., China, Nux
v., a/o
Indication: Liver diseases
Available as: Tablets (50 pcs.),
ampules (5 pcs. 1.1 ml ea.)

Husteel (Heel)
Ingredients: Ars.j., Bell., Scilla,
Cupr.-ac., Caust.
Indication: Cough, colds
Available as: Drops [1 oz. (30 ml)]

Leptandra compositum (Heel)
Ingredients: Lept., Podo., Carp.-v.,
Phos., a/o
Indication: Liver and pancreatic
disorders
Available as: Drops [1 oz. (30 ml)],
ampules (4 pcs., 2.2 ml ea.)

Lymphomyosot (Heel)
Ingredients: Myosotis arvensis,
Veronica, Teucr., a/o

Indication: Tonsillitis, glandular
swelling (e.g., thyroid)
Available as: Drops [1 oz. (30 ml)]
ampules (5 pcs., 1.1 ml ea.)

Mercurius-Heel (Heel)
Ingredients : Merc., Hep., Lach.,
Phyt., Bell.
Indication: Tonsillitis, catarrh,
suppurative diseases
Available as: Tablets (50 pcs.)

Nux vomica-Homaccord (Heel)
Ingredients: Nux-v., Bry., Lyc.,
Coloc.
Indication: Diseases of the diges-
tive tract, constipation, poisoning
Available as: Drops [1 oz. (30 ml)],
ampules (5 pcs., 1.1 ml ea.)

Oculoheel (Heel)
Ingredients: Apis, Rhus.-t., Hep.,
Spig., Staph., a/o
Indication: Inflammation of the
eyes
Available as: Tablets (50 pcs.)

Osteoheel (Heel)
Ingredients: Hekla, Kali.-j., Aran.,
Nat.-s., Calc.-p., a/o
Indication: Bone diseases
Available as: Tablets (50 pcs.)

Phosphor-Homaccord (Heel)
Ingredients: Phos., Arg.-n., Par.
Indication: Pharyngitis,
pneumonia
Available as: Tablets (50 pcs.)

Plantago-Homaccord (Heel)
Ingredients: Plan., Bell., Ingn.
Indication: Cystitis
Available as: Drops [1 oz. (30 ml)]
ampules (5 pcs. 1.1 ml ea.)

Reneel (Heel)
Indication: Berb., Canth., Pareir.,
Caust., a/o
Indication: Nephritis, cystitis,
urinary calculi
Available as: Tablets (50 pcs.)

Schwef-Heel (Heel)
Ingredients: Sulfur
Indication: Skin disorders, eczema
Available as: Drops [1 oz. (30 ml)]

Solidago compositum S (Heel)
Ingredients: Solid., Berb., Hep.,
Caps., a/o
Indication: Acute and chronic
urinary disorders, urinary sediment, calculi
Available as: Ampules (4 pcs., 2.2
ml ea.)

Spascupreel (Heel)
Ingredients: Coloc., Am.-b., Atro.,
Verat., Gels., a/o
Indication: Colic, spasms (e.g.,
intestines, urethra)
Available as: Tablets (50 pcs.),
ampules (5 pcs., 1.1 ml ea.), suppositories (12 pcs., 2 g ea.)

Sulfur-Heel (Heel)
Ingredients: Sulf., Mez., Calad., a/o
Indication: Skin disorders, eczema
Available as: Tablets (50 pcs.)

Traumeel (Heel)
Ingredients: Arn., Calend., Ham.,
Bell., Acon., a/o
Indication: All types of injuries

Available as: Tablets (50 pcs.),
drops [1 oz. (30 ml)], ampules (4
pcs., 2.2 ml ea.), ointment (50 g)

Viropect (DHU)
Ingredients: Ip., Dros., Cupr.-ac.,
Indication: Cough spasm
Available as: Powder (2 g)

Bach Flowers

All 38 Bach Flowers, as well as the
emergency drops (Rescue-Drops)
are available without presciption
in all homeopathic pharmacies, in
most health food stores, and
through mail order services. They
are available in 10-ml vials, which
are the mother tinctures, and the
Rescue drops are also available in
20-ml vials. You can also get Bach
Flower essences in combination
formulations (available in alcohol,
water, and in vinegar).

Agrimony
Agrimonia eupatoria
Indication: Restlessness,
contrariness

Aspen
Populus tremula
Indication: Fear of the unknown,
fear at night

Beech
Fagus sylvatica
Indication: Easily put off, hair
stands up

Centaury
Centaurium erythrea
(C. umbellatum)
Indication: Submissive to receive
affection

Cerato
Ceratostigma willmottiana
Indication: Indecision, insecurity

Cherry Plum
Prunus cerasifera
Indication: Impulsive violence,
wide-eyed anger, dilated pupils

Chestnut Bud
Aesculus hippocastanum
Indication: Repeats the same
mistakes

Glossary

Allopathy
A system of medicinal practice involving use of medicines that produce effects different from those of the disease treated; in principle, the opposite of homeopathy. This term is erroneously used for the regular practice of medicine by physicians.

Anthropozoonosis
An infectious disease that is naturally transmissible between humans and animals (e.g., rabies, salmonellosis, ringworm).

Antibiotic Susceptibility Test
A laboratory method that involves testing microorganisms for resistance to antibiotics and to determine those antibiotics which are effective and at what dosage.

Aspiration Puncture
Puncturing a fluid-filled tissue (cyst, abscess, hematoma), for the purpose of removing the liquid.

Aujeszky's Disease
Also called Pseudo-rabies; a viral disease characterized by salivation, itching, vomiting, and paralysis. An acute and fatal disease.

Borreliosis
Tick-borne relapsing fever. Incubation period from 3 to 12 days or longer. Begins with flu-like symptoms, continues into paralytic episodes.

Calculi
Stone formation in the kidney or bladder, usually composed of mineral salts.

Callus
New bone formation at the site of a fracture.

Carrier
An animal that carries and sheds infectious agents, without showing symptoms of disease.

Castration (Spaying/Neutering)
Surgical removal of the gonads: ovaries in the female and testes in the male.

Chlamydia
Bacteria-like infectious agents which cause eye and nose infections.

Combination Remedy
A homeopathic remedy that is composed of a number of single remedy substances.

Constitution
The overall condition—physical, psychological, and mental—of an individual. This includes the tendency of this individual to contract certain disorders.

Constitutional Remedy
A remedy that is targeted at an individual's overall physical and psychological body character to initiate its own healing processes.

Diabetes
Disorder of the glucose metabolism due to lack of insulin. It leads to accumulation of sugar in the blood and urine.

Disposition
A natural tendency toward acquiring a certain disorder.

Ectoparasite
A parasite that invades the external surface of the animal, either temporarily or permanently.

Edema, Edematous
Accumulation of tissue fluids, leading to swelling.

Electrolyte
A substance which, in solution, contains positively and negatively charged particles (e.g., acids, bases, salts).

Endoparasite
A parasite that invades and lives inside the organism of another animal.

Euthanasia
Humane killing with the support of an anesthetic.

Feline AIDS
An incurable feline viral infectious disease, which is resistant to any current therapeutics.

Feline Leukemia
Viral infection that destroys the white blood cell system, leading to death.

FIP
Acronym for Feline Infectious Peritonitis. A viral infectious disease of the lining of the body cavities.

Gastritis
Inflammation or ulceration of the stomach.

Hemolysis
Breakdown of the red blood cells.

Immune Serum
Serum that contains antibodies and can be used to fight infectious diseases.

Incubation Period
Interval between the time of infection and the appearance of symptoms.

Mother tincture
Remedies from the vegetable world are processed under strict criteria, and converted into a liquid form, the mother tincture.

Mycotic dermatitis (dermatophytosis)
Fungal infection of the skin.

Palpation
Examining a diseased area by touching.

Pathogen
A microorganism capable of producing disease.

Phlegmon
A suppurative inflammation under the skin.

Pyometra
Retained pus accumulation in the uterus.

Rabies
A fatal viral infection that is transmissible between humans and animals. Symptoms are salivation, spasms, gagging, and paralysis (near death).

Resorption
Tissue absorbs a substance that is administered in the form of a solution.

Rickets
Form of bone deformation in kittens due to lack of vitamin D, and insufficient lime deposits in developing bones.

Rolly Season
Colloquial synonym for a cat in heat.

Septicemia
A severe systemic infection, usually characterized by high fever.

Single Remedy
A homeopathic remedy which contains a single homeopathic substance.

Spores
Progeny of plant cells and fungi.

Sterilization
Rendering an animal barren. Surgical interruption of the vas deferens (male) or the uterine tubes (female). The gonads remain in the animal. Hormones continue to be produced, and sexual drive is intact.

Suppurative
Producing or associated with production of pus.

Toxoplasmosis
A disease caused by a one-cell organism that may be carried by a cat without symptoms of disease. It is transmissible to humans. The symptoms and signs of the human disease are fever, diarrhea, paralysis, gastroenteritis, and meningitis.

Uremia
The blood is poisoned by urinary components.

Index of Health Problems

Useful Literature

● Bach, Edward, *Heal Thyself. An Explanation of the Real Cause and Cure of Disease.* The C. W. Daniel Company Ltd., 1931.

● – – –, *The Twelve Healers.* The C. W. Daniel Company Ltd., 1933.

● Chancellor, Philip M., (ed.), *Handbook of the Bach Flower Remedies.* The C. W. Daniel Company Ltd., 1971.

● de Bairacli-Levy, Juliette, *The Complete Herbal Handbook for the Dog and Cat.* Arco Publishing, New York, 1991.

● Harper, Joan, *The Healthy Cat and Dog Cookbook.* E.P. Dutton, New York.

● Howard, Judy, *Bach Flower Remedies Step by Step.* The C. W. Daniel Company Ltd., 1990.

● Howard, Judy, *Story of Mount Vernon.* Mount Vernon, Oxford, 1986.

● Howard, Judy and Ramsell, John, *The Original Writings of Edward Bach, Curators and Trustees.* The C. W. Daniel Company Ltd., 1990.

● Jones, T. W. Hyne, *Dictionary of the Bach F lower Remedies, Positive and Negative Aspects.* The C. W. Daniel Company Ltd., 1976.

● Pitcairn, Richard H., DVM, and Susan Hubble Pitcairn, *Natural Health Care for Dogs and Cats.* Rodale Press, Emmaus, PA.

● Ramsell, John, *Questions and Answers Clarifying the Basic Principles and Standards of the Bach Flower Remedies.* Mount Vernon. Mount Vernon, Oxford, 1986.

● Stein, Diane, *Natural Healing for Dogs and Cats.* Crossing Press, Freedom, CA, 1993.

● Vithoulkas, George, *The Science of Homeopathy.* Random House, Inc., New York, 1980.

● Weeks/Bullen, *Bach Flower Remedies Illustrations and Preparations.* The C. W. Daniel Company Ltd., 1964.

● Wheeler, F.J., MRCS, LRCP. *The Bach Remedies Repertory, A supplementary guide to the use of herbal remedies discovered by Edward Bach.* The C. W. Daniel Company Ltd., London, 1952.

Useful Addresses

● American Holistic Veterinarian Medical Association
2214 Old Emmorton Road
Bel Air, MD 21015
(410) 569-0795 (nationwide referrals)

● International Veterinarian Acupuncture Society
c/o Meredith Snader, DVM
Executive Director
RD #4, Box 216
Chester Springs, PA 19425
(215) 827-7245

● International Foundation for Homeopathy
2366 Eastlake Avenue E.
Suite 301
Seattle, WA 98102
(206) 324-8230

● National Center for Homeopathy
801 North Fairfax Street, Suite 306
Alexandria, VA 22314
(703) 548-7790

● Nelson Bach, USA, Ltd.
Wilmington Technology Park
100 Research Drive
Wilmington, MA 01887-4406
(800) 334-0843

The Author

Rudolf Deiser, DVM, has worked as a clinical veterinarian since 1979. He passed the boards in Natural Health Care in 1989. He treats most small animal patients according to holistic medical methods. Since 1990 he has also treated human patients with classic homeopathic remedies.

Publishing Information

Published originally under the title *Naturheilpraxis HUNDE*
© 1996 by Grafe und Unzer Verlag GmbH, München
English translation © Copyright 1997 by Barron's Educational Series, Inc.

All inquiries should be addressed to:
Barron's Educational Series, Inc.
250 Wireless Boulevard
Hauppauge, New York 11788

Library of Congress Catalog Card No. 97-15620

International Standard Book Number 0-7641-0123-4

Library of Congress Cataloging-in-Publication Data
Deiser, Rudolf.
    [Naturheil praxis Katzen.   English]
    Natural health care for your cat / Rudolf Deiser.
       p.   cm.
    Includes bibliographical references and index.
    ISBN 0-7641-0123-4
      1. Cats. 2. Cats—Health. 3. Cats—Diseases—Alternative
treatment. I. Title.
    SF447.D5313   1997
    636.8'0896024—dc21   97-15620
                                            CIP

Printed in Hong Kong
9 8 7 6 5 4 3 2 1

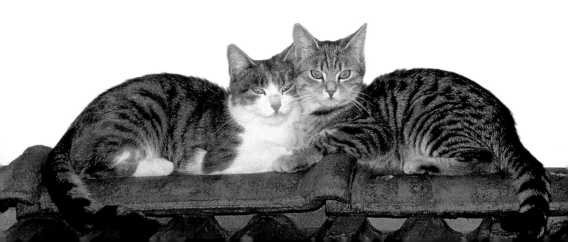